The Promised Landing
A Gateway to Peaceful Dying

Bart Windrum

2018

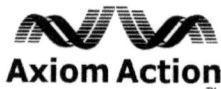

Other books by Bart Windrum

Notes from the Waiting Room:
Managing a Loved One's End-of-Life Hospitalization

How to Efficiently Settle the Family Estate

Bart Windrum is available for speaking engagements and workshops
Bart@AxiomAction.com
Obtain other contact information at AxiomAction.com

The Promised Landing: A Gateway to Peaceful Dying
Copyright ©2018 Bart Windrum. All rights reserved.

No part of this book may be used, reproduced, or stored in any manner whatsoever without the publisher's written permission, except in the case of brief quotations used with attribution in articles or reviews.

The content of this book is based upon the author's personal experience and inquiry. This book does not provide medical or legal advice. This book is not intended as a substitute for professional medical guidance or professional legal guidance. The author and publisher are not responsible for any adverse effects or consequences resulting from the use of information or opinions contained within this book. The author and publisher assume no responsibility for errors, omissions, or inconsistencies.

Publisher's Cataloging-In-Publication Data
The promised landing: a gateway to peaceful dying / Bart Windrum.
viii, 216, 23cm
ISBN   978-0-9801090-4-7
ISBN   978-0-9801090-5-4   eBook
1. Death—Terminology 2. Death—Psychological aspects 3. Death—Planning
I. Title II. Author   PE1599.D4
Library of Congress Control Number: 2017916996

Book Design, Cover Design, Graphics: Bart Windrum
Typefaces: Trajan Pro, Stone Serif, Stone Sans
54 color graphic images
Technical production consulting: Jay Nelson
Author photographs: rap, Dave McCollum; portrait, Will Eiserman

1 3.18   2 5.18

For Jadrienne Windrum

For those who have the sense
that the implied promise of conventional end-of-life guidance
leaves too much unaddressed,
and who want to keep their own end-of-life promise
to die in peace, and at peace.

Contents

Why

Lexicon	3
Glide Path	4
Is This Book for You?	5
Getting to Peace	7
Understanding Demises as Destinations Within Our Dying Territory	11
Promises, Promises	23
Glossary of Thoughts	29
Impetus	31

Our Dying Territory:
Identifying and Naming our Dying Situations

Chapter 1	Matrix Underpinnings: Promises and Practicalities	34
Chapter 2	Matrix Genesis: A Zillion Words for Snow	39
Chapter 3	Matrix Basics: Cardinal Aspects	44
Chapter 4	Matrix Territory: Where're You Gonna Land?	50
Chapter 5	Matrix Time-out	52
Chapter 6	Matrix: Landings	56
Chapter 7	Matrix: Ethics and Legalities	78
Chapter 8	Matrix: Landing Vignettes	83
Chapter 9	Matrix: Guided Recitation	102

Obstacles to Peaceful Dying and How to Mitigate Them

Chapter 10	To Die in Peace: Our Rights of Passage	126
1	Difficulty distinguishing among dying situations	130
2	Trouble determining when enough is enough	131
3	Over-reliance on advance directives	134
•	Obstacles 1–3 Reflection	137
4	Exposure to medical snafus (misadventures and/or errors)	139
5	Ignorance regarding life-support matters including systemic overrides	141
6	Inability to advocate medically for a loved one or oneself	145
•	Obstacles 4–6 Reflection	147
7	The Opaque Dying Marketplace	149
•	To Die in Peace: Our Rights of Passage Recap	167
•	Our 21st Century End-of-life Milieu	169
Chapter 11	Deus Ex Machina?	170

And So

Appendix A	The Rusted Gate	174
Appendix B	Never Say Die Rap	176
Appendix C	On Advocating	178
	Independent Thinker, No One's Rube	178
	Can't Touch the Sky	180
	Call 911 When It's Time to Pass?	185
	If You Don't Talk You Don't Get No Say	187
	No Bro Ma'am You Ain't Goin' Nowhere	192
	Study Up, Make Some Sense	198
Appendix D	Matrix Visual History	202
Appendix E	The Quickie Button	205
Appendix F	Coming In and Speaking Out	207

Acknowledgments   208
Index   214

Why

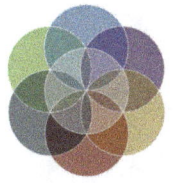

Lexicon

My mother's unexpected hospitalized demise during January 2004 and my father's error-caused demise during the spring of 2005 were unnecessarily painful events for our family. In response, I became activated and developed an end-of-life body of work to help each of us achieve the peaceful deaths to which we aspire. This lexicon—a set of insights and assessments describing a worldview—identifies personal and systematized obstacles to peaceful dying and how we may mitigate them.

From 2005 through 2008 I authored *Notes from the Waiting Room: Managing a Loved One's End-of-Life Hospitalization* and *How to Effectively Settle the Family Estate*. During 2012–2013, I presented a TEDx talk, "To Die in Peace: New Terms of Engagement"; wrote, arranged, and performed the "Never Say Die Rap"; published the article, "It's Time to Account for Medical Error in 'Top Ten Causes of Death' Charts" in the *Journal of Participatory Medicine*; and created a unique end-of-life visioning tool, "Windrum's Matrix of Dying Terms."

Windrum's Matrix is this book's primary focus. The Matrix names the array of dying situations ahead of us. It frames them as our *dying territory* containing destinations that we can learn to aim toward and, as importantly, aim to avoid.

In 2014 I completed the lexicon, formalizing it as a program and naming it "To Die in Peace: Our Rights of Passage." Windrum's Matrix is the entrance to the program.

The Promised Landing serves as a gateway and as a guide to the entire lexicon.

Chart your glide path while there's time
to die in peace with minimal cryin'
Study up, make some sense
of 21st century impediments
Time to grow up before we get old
There's more to dying than we've been told
Wishing won't help us turn the page
So 17 new terms to engage
I have a Matrix for that...

— from the *Never Say Die Rap*

Is This Book for You?

Have you endured, during the demise of a loved one, circumstances so distressing that you are determined to never experience a situation like that again? Are you worried that deaths of loved ones in the foreseeable future may play out contrary to what they, and you, prefer?

Do you wonder if what you have done, or have yet to do, regarding the end of your own life will be sufficient to increase your likelihood of dying in peace?

Do you question how to protect yourself and your family from pressures that escalate dying into a technological battle against death despite its obvious nearness? Are you concerned that you and your loved ones might be among those responsible for such a situation?

Are you confident that the promises you've heard, assumed, or made to yourself for a peaceful death will be fulfilled?

Are you certain that spiritual engagement will suffice to protect you from end-of-life outcomes you hope to avoid?

Even if your family has filled out advance directive documents and engaged in conversations about end-of-life matters, do these apprehensions persist?

Are you interested in taking a deep, sustained look at the obstacles arrayed between you and your desire to die in peace?

Are you willing to apply additional effort to learn how to mitigate or even overcome those obstacles?

If you suspect that there's more to dying than we've been told, if you want to make some sense of 21st century impediments, if you discern that wishing won't really help and are ready for something that will, this book is for you.

The Promised Landing opens a gateway to peaceful dying. It presents a solution for a prevalent yet previously unidentified problem: our inability to differentiate among common dying situations. I'll name and describe every dying situation we experience in today's world. We will see all of them combined as our dying territory, where the different dying situations are way stations and destinations that we can learn to aim for, and aim to avoid.

To accomplish this, I have developed a tool that names our dying situations: Windrum's Matrix of Dying Terms. *The Promised Landing* presents the Matrix element by element, culminating in a spoken recitation through which we will take a personal tour of our dying territory, imaginatively placing ourselves throughout it. We'll then locate our dying territory within the larger context of other significant obstacles to peaceful dying which, taken together, comprise a practical end-of-life lexicon, To Die in Peace: Our Rights of Passage. The Matrix and the lexicon will function as a gateway for your further exploration of what is required, of each of us, to die in peace and at peace.

If you have not yet considered dying matters or your own future death, if you have not yet been rattled by a loved one's troubling demise, this book will still serve you. Depending upon your constitution, you may feel a bit challenged; *The Promised Landing* is not introductory-level material according to conventionally presented end-of-life discussions, although from my perspective it starts at exactly the right place.

The Promised Landing also offers medical professionals new language to help guide the patients and families they serve toward more peaceful dying.

Getting to Peace

I might experience peaceful dying.
I might experience peace-less dying.
How about you?

How about giving voice to these possibilities? Say out loud, with deliberate emphasis although not over-emphasis:

"I might experience peace-less dying."
"I might experience peaceful dying."

Does voicing these possibilities activate any mental response, emotions, or even physical sensations? Does doing so increase or decrease your confidence in achieving the death you want and avoiding the type of death you would prefer not to experience?

If you've filled out advance directive documents and assigned a proxy to represent you should the need arise, does having done these things offer clues about how to obtain the outcome you want and avoid the one you don't want? If you've engaged in spiritual development focused on end-of-life outcomes, does it feel sufficient for achieving the kind of death you'd prefer?

The Promised Landing is about identifying and mitigating obstacles to dying in peace. Obstacles peculiar to our time await all of us throughout our dying territory. When we become ensnared by them (most of us do…), we suffer from stressors and risks in addition to those inherent in dying. We can learn to identify, recognize, and plan around these obstacles before we're upon them and they are upon us. Because the obstacles, by definition, infringe on peace, this is not a book about peace; it's a book about *getting to peace*. *The Promised Landing: A Gateway to Peaceful Dying* points the way toward peaceful end-of-life experiences.

"Toward" means that it will take us all some doing to get there. The first step is to pass through a gateway, stepping through a rarely used gate.

A gateway is a means toward achieving a state or condition. In the physical world, gateways rise over and frame gates. A gateway makes a gate into a statement, imparting importance to the passage, letting us know that something substantial awaits us on the other side. Metaphorically, the end-of-life gate before us is rusted from disuse. This rusted gate may take some effort to open. It may squeak and squeal, and so may we. We might not like everything we encounter as we step through into a space we've purposefully avoided for most, if not all, of our lives. We may need to occasionally take a mental and emotional breath, find our equilibrium, as we traverse the place. It's a place known by an anti-name: *death denial*. And traverse it we must; one step doesn't get us very far.

As we wend our way through our dying territory, we will become *death-literate*—knowledgeable about matters pertaining to forces shaping, if not controlling, our dying time. I can promise that you will increase your likelihood of dying in peace by making this journey.

In our death-denying and medicalized culture, only the fortunate few, graced with great luck or good fortune, attain a peaceful demise without arduous effort. For most of us, finding our promised landing will require a new response to how we personally approach and manage dying—through attention, openness, study, and preparation. This is what is meant by death literacy.

Except for the considerable emotional toll extracted by needlessly hard deaths common to those who remain death-illiterate, death denial is easy. All it requires is our refusal to address end-of-life matters. Death literacy requires us to face the end-of-life problems we have made for ourselves—now, well before our dying time, while we're otherwise busy living our lives. Increasing our likelihood of dying in peace requires us to understand the personal and systemic obstacles between us and our end-of-life promises. It requires us to recognize that by doing nothing now (death denial), we reinforce the likelihood of our last weeks and days on planet Earth being overly stressful and peace-less.

Medicine's repeated message is that filling out advance directives and appointing an advocate will result in peaceful dying. And many people hope that spiritual engagement will provide a bulwark against the strong socio-medical tide carrying millions of us to protracted, overmedicalized deaths. My experiences have taught me that more is required. We must learn to identify, understand, and manage a range of prevalent obstacles standing between our desire for peaceful deaths and the types of deaths that too many of our loved ones have experienced—deaths which millions of us have witnessed, or participated in, and reject as inhumane.

Our challenges arise largely from opacity around end-of-life matters. Our medical system too often, if not typically, withholds end-of-life information from us and sugar-coats what little it is willing to voice. So we deny and medicine obscures; we're unused to taking a long and serious look at factors inhibiting a peaceful glide path at the end of our lives. *The Promised Landing* offers a sustained serious look.

I strive to address the topic in terms of likelihoods, not certainties. One truth I can declare with certainty is this: we who do not deal with matters of how we die while healthy and living will deal with them, for the very first time, while sick and dying. For those who wait, the emotional toll for all involved will be profoundly deeper than for those who choose to become death literate in advance of dying. Doing so may feel disquieting at first but will be gratifying when you know, in your heart and in your bones, that the effort you exert now has resulted in the knowledge and familiarity required to increase your chances of obtaining the dying experience that you or your loved ones would prefer.

Increasing our likelihood of peaceful dying does not guarantee a trouble-free demise, but it's the best we can do and worth doing well. By minimizing the likelihood of infringement due to obstacles built into our socio-medical system, we open emotional and soul space throughout a demise to make peace with intrinsic aspects of dying—our plain human experiences and relations.

Be patient on your journey through *The Promised Landing*. The obstacle to dying in peace that Windrum's Matrix describes and solves, despite its prevalence, will seem unfamiliar. It takes some time to explain. Reading this book may feel like making an odyssey. *This is a working voyage.* As with any long trip, we'll begin by considering where we're starting from and imagine where we're going. We'll orient ourselves, unfold a new map, learn to read it, and explore the unknown. We'll see new sights and learn the landmarks; the unfamiliar will become familiar as we name situations that we may have already experienced but haven't thought to name or formalize. Eventually the stimuli will coalesce into a new way of perceiving our end-of-life experiences. As our death denial fog lifts, our dying territory and obstacles to successfully navigating it will emerge as a new landscape. Viewing that horizon, we'll be better positioned to chart our glide paths to the peaceful dying experiences we want.

Many potential obstacles, and variations on obstacles, infringe on dying in peace. Considering them all will require engagement beyond this book (see Study Up, Make Some Sense at the end of Appendix C). *The Promised Landing* focuses on common, ever-present aspects of late-life medical encounters that deliver profound and often unwanted consequences. It does not directly address other obstacles such as insurance coverage shenanigans; religious influences; social inequities; end-of-life politicization; spiritual development; extra-legal self-deliverance; matters of long declines; aging in place; or finding, obtaining, and paying for late-life services. Its lessons will serve as underpinnings for choices you make about these matters.

Welcome to my world... may your visit here improve yours.

Understanding Demises as Destinations Within Our Dying Territory

The following stories of three demises introduce and set the context for exploring our dying territory. My parents' unexpected terminal hospitalizations exemplify two of the harder end-of-life landings. How one doctor adapted this work's message when counseling a dying patient's family exemplifies its utility for medical professionals.

At the end of each story, I will introduce new terms that name the situations described. These new terms may make sense, or they may raise questions. In either case, know that chapters 1–9 will fully explain the terms, their meaning, and what they represent in our lives, our deaths, and our memories.

As a prelude, here's a glimpse into the vibrant life my parents led before stumbling into their dying territory.

The Good Years: 1970 Through the Early 2000s

In 1970 my parents, Ruth and Mort Greenberg, then empty nesters, changed careers, leaving bookkeeping, aluminum railing manufacturing, and Florida. They borrowed $5,000 from Mom's parents, Rose and Max Logue, to buy a Sir Speedy Instant Printing retail franchise on East Colfax Avenue in Denver, Colorado. It was the dawn of a new service known as quick printing, the first time that people could obtain high-quality copies in a few minutes from a storefront business. Fifteen years before the introduction of the first personal computers, while-you-wait short-run printing was a real convenience.

They worked hard—I know because I worked with them for seven years doing counter sales and delivery; bindery; and typesetting, pasteup, and layout. They built a business from scratch at ages 47 and 50 and retired 15 years later with enough earned and saved to comfortably live out their remaining lives.

Mom was a contest winner in the days when limerick and cooking contests were the rage. Dad was a former electrical engineer who had professionally designed the first color television kit. As a print shop proprietor, he became as outgoing as Mom, enjoying their customers, who appreciated him in return. In that less politically correct time, Dad designed pin-on buttons reading: "How About a Quickie At Sir Speedy?," which he handed out to everybody, male and female, who entered the store. He'd offer the button while asking with a twinkle, "Would you like a Quickie?" Virtually everybody appreciated the clever wordplay; most people in fact had come for a while-you-wait "quick-print" order, and asking if a print job was a while-you-wait (typically 25 to 100 resumes) or drop-off (for example, 3000 8.5" x 5.5" three-part carbonless forms printed two-up, sliced, and padded) was our first question of customers. I have the sole remaining Quickie button pinned in my office. When I asked Dad years later how he changed from taciturn engineer to outgoing guy he said, simply and cryptically, "I changed my face."

Years before the 1985 release of Microsoft® Excel, Mort hired a software programmer to create a customized spreadsheet on which he ran countless business scenarios at night. He became known throughout the national Sir Speedy community for achieving the highest profit margin of any store. We constantly combined and re-queued print orders to maximize efficiency back at the presses, which required time-consuming adjustments for different paper stocks, ink coverage, and colors. Ruth was so accurate with the store's books that one year, an auditing Colorado Department of Revenue agent over-analyzed them for days, suspecting that Mom's perfection was covering up some malfeasance.

A significant fraction of Sir Speedy's traffic was for business cards. To capture the revenue lost by sending out for popular raised-letter cards, my parents started ThermoPrint, a companion business printing raised-letter stationary, in a space around the corner from Sir Speedy. We used to dash between both print shops via the shared courtyard behind each space, the shortest route between them.

After 15 years, the folks sold both stores. The day after fulfilling his two-week post-sale commitment to help the new owners come up to speed, the very first day of his retirement, Mort suffered a heart attack with multiple cardiac arrests. Mom and I witnessed his resuscitation via electroshock paddles. That day he received his first of two double cardiac bypasses. Medicine did well by him and for us; he lived another 19 years.

Ruth and Mort obtained a modest motorhome and spent a portion of many years traveling the United States and Canada. Eventually they moved to south Florida's Atlantic seaboard where numerous relatives had previously settled. My parents remained outgoing in their post-retirement, but starting in her mid-70s, Mom's interest in the grist of life diminished. She played computer solitaire but never learned to use email. She left it to Dad, despite his deteriorating mobility, to walk their little dog. And Dad didn't realize until after her death that most of the doctors' appointments on their calendar were for her, not him—a surprise since he was the one with mounting comorbidities from a type-A personality, the two cardiac bypasses, high blood pressure, diabetes, and a poorly executed hip replacement that eventually necessitated a redo, a walker, and a motorized scooter. Aside from slowing down, Mom's apparently minor medical problems were insignificant compared to Dad's. Or so we thought...

January 2004
Suspended Dying, under Machine control
within the Medically managed Progressed timeframe

At age 81, while in a hospital lobby awaiting an outpatient appointment, Mom experienced sudden respiratory distress. Dad was elsewhere in the facility. Mom accepted emergency medical aid and was almost instantly intubated—placed on a breathing machine. Dad called us in tears from the intensive care unit (ICU), and the next day my sister and I arrived at its door in south Florida from our homes in the Denver metropolitan area.

In 2004 we were what I've come to call "dying newbies." We were a small family; just the four of us. My parents had shared their advance directives with us, and we'd had several family conversations about end-of-life matters. My sister Judy, a newborn intensive care unit (NICU) nurse, was technically knowledgeable yet unprepared, as were Dad and I, for what turned out to be a callous medical environment. And there we were, all of us fully expecting Dad to have dropped dead first, staring at Ruth, who was unconscious with a depressed internal temperature and "wired up" in the chilly ICU under only a thin top sheet. She was later described to me as the sickest patient in the facility at that time.

Mom remained in critical condition on machine ventilation for over two weeks until efforts to save her proved futile. I never thought to ask Dad if that is what they had wanted. We were all just shocked. Those endless days were emotionally brutal, filled with care-lessness, clinical errors, ineffective treatment handoffs (referred to as "discontinuity" in the medical profession), hard surroundings, and the adverse mismanagement of communication with our patient-family. I detail the many lessons we learned there in my first book, *Notes from the Waiting Room: Managing a Loved One's End-of-Life Hospitalization*.

My family experienced a particular type of dying situation. We had no name for it at the time. I've since named it, along with 16 others. All dying situations are identifiable if we reflect upon their timing, and who or what exerts predominant control over our decline and then our final days (referred to as active dying). At the time of Mom's collapse, she landed in a place I now call *Delayed* dying, her death being delayed by the introduction of life-support equipment. During those weeks, we all traversed Mom's dying territory, ending up in a situation I call *Suspended* dying. That designation derives from the writing of medical anthropologist Sharon Kaufman who, in her book *And a Time to Die: How American Hospitals Shape the End of Life*, identified a state peculiar to our time: an indeterminate state, neither living nor dying, suspended between the two. In this state, the ventilator machine was doing Mom's breathing for her; it was the prominent aspect of our experience throughout her demise. Her treatment was highly medically managed, and the course of her disease extended well beyond its onset, into what medicine calls a Progressed timeframe. Adding these aspects together, in the language of Windrum's Matrix of Dying Terms, we experienced Suspended dying, under Machine control, at the Progressed stage of a Medically managed demise. Those are all the parameters; I simply say Suspended dying for short.

If you've had the misfortune to be a surrogate for a dying loved one or to attend a loved one's demise under these circumstances, you probably understand that "Suspended" is an apt descriptor for both the dying and the living during such a dying experience.

Kaufman identified and described my patient-family's experience of Mom's demise perfectly. Dad's death 15 months later was another sort entirely.

April–May 2005
Erroneous Dying, under Medical control within the
Abrupt timeframe... devolving to Endstate Dying within the
Medically managed Endstage timeframe

After a year's mourning, at age 84 Dad sold their condominium and moved into a brand new assisted-living apartment in a continuum-of-care community. He liked watching the world go by on the heavily trafficked road beyond the grounds. He drove off to lunch every day, steering a motorized "scooter" to his van, winching it into its bay, toddling to the driver's seat, then tooling off like the highly skilled driver he was. Within a month he realized that neither his aged cousins nor my middle-aged cousins who lived nearby were close enough family to see him through his closing years. He took interest in returning to Colorado to finish his days near my sister, myself, and my wife and daughter. Since he'd been living at sea level for seven years and only one-third of his heart muscle was functional after the bypass operations, we discussed his options while hoping fervently that he could return to mile-high Colorado and its thin, less-oxygenated air. I especially looked forward to hosting Dad in the iconic compact city I live in, nestled against Colorado's Front Range.

The default medical pathway at the time was to test for cardiac pacemaker eligibility and to implant one if he were found eligible. Treadmill stress testing was out of the question, so a nuclear stress test was ordered. Radioactive dye introduced intravenously would reveal the state of his heart at rest and then under the stress induced by stimulating the heart with another intravenous medication. I never heard mention of risk, nor was Dad advised that the test could prove disastrous; it was presented to us as the "standard of care." In our conversations, we never thought to discuss its advisability, and I never heard or thought to ask questions related to failing the test. As far as I know, his cardiologist never offered the possibility of using oxygen as a non-invasive option. To this day I do not know if supplemental oxygen might have been viable. Recently, a cardiologist reminded me that many people with Dad's troubles live their lives at mile-high elevation; that his transition back might have been possible with the assistance of bottled oxygen.

I will always regret that we weren't smart enough to have investigated alternatives. Dad rolled the dice and lost. His overly-stressed heart medically "crashed" during the test and he wound up admitted to a major medical center on the south Florida Atlantic seaboard. I received the call while on a windsurfing vacation in South Padre Island, Texas, stowed my gear, parked the SUV, and flew to Florida.

Shortly after Judy and I arrived, Dad acquired, through a urinary catheter, a preventable, hospital-caused, often fatal "superbug" infection—methicillin-resistant Staphylococcus aureus (MRSA). The infection migrated to his bloodstream; one eventual and acute effect was a ballooned wrist on his dominant hand causing debilitating pain.

Delirium set in and Dad's demise played out over a two-week hospitalization. It took the doctors a week to identify his swollen wrist as infected. During that time, he could not use his primary hand and the other arm held the IV lines, so his ability to manipulate objects, including his hearing aids, was severely compromised. He had gone unfed for several days; we had to hire help to be there to feed him.

Despite having begun the long process of reflecting on our experiences during Mom's demise, Judy and I were still far from knowledgeable proxies, and many hard lessons were in store for us (these, too, detailed in *Notes from the Waiting Room*). Problems similar to those we'd experienced during Mom's terminal hospitalization the prior year arose, but we failed to recognize them because the nature of Dad's medical conditions differed from Mom's. We weren't yet attuned to the systemic nature of the obstacles to dying in peace.

The facility was better than where Mom died, but that didn't preclude repeat shocks and harm, including some of our most bitter lessons regarding advance directives and supposed personal agency. Dad didn't agree to the Do-Not-Resuscitate Order (DNR) override that would have been imposed upon him had he undergone the short surgery to drain the wrist infection under general anesthesia; his doctors required the override given his many medical conditions, but he didn't want to end up like Mom. I wouldn't learn for 18 months that we could have been offered a "time-based" option limiting the use of life supports post-surgery. We might have taken that risk as the only hope for restoring him (itself probably futile, as was the dubious choice for an 84-year-old with all Dad's conditions undergoing the nuclear pacemaker test in the first place). But we were given no options. Dad admitted himself to the in-hospital hospice wing (itself a troublesome process) and died there several days later. Due to further snafus affecting the way his demise played out, I never had a closing goodbye conversation with my father—an absence that haunts me no matter how many years pass. Painful regret and grief arise anew whenever I find myself revisiting this.

In the new language of Windrum's Matrix of Dying Terms, we experienced *Erroneous* dying under Medical control. My family's and the doctor's errors in judgement and the MRSA infection were the related causes.* Over 10 days' time, we traversed Dad's dying territory, starting from medical error in the Abrupt timeframe and landing in *Endstate* dying within the Endstage timeframe. His last four days, in hospice, were too short a time to qualify as *Collaborative* dying.

October 2015
One Doctor's Experience of Our Dying Territory

Until October 2015 my end-of-life presentations had been general, summarizing my entire lexicon, too brief to fully explain any part of it. That month, I presented my first workshop devoted solely to exploring our dying territory using Windrum's Matrix of Dying Terms, at an end-of-life conference in Los Angeles, California.

---

*Two aspects of my father's catheter-associated urinary tract infection (CAUTI) require explanation to clarify why I classify his death as medically Erroneous.

The attending registered nurse used a wrong-sized urinary catheter. Upon insertion Dad yelped. The RN subsequently acknowledged not having the right size at hand. This poor medical practice, not considered in and of itself to be medical error, introduces potentially adverse outcomes. My father, who had never had a UTI in his life, experienced a direct, ultimately fatal outcome.

The U.S. Centers for Medicare & Medicaid Services (CMS) maintains a list of "serious, preventable, and costly" hospital-acquired conditions ("never events") that it says ought not to occur. CMS penalizes hospitals by adjusting or withholding payment for subsequent treatments that mitigating the conditions require. CAUTIs are a listed condition. See www.cms.gov/Medicare/Medicare-Fee-for-Service-Payment/HospitalAcqCond/Hospital-Acquired_Conditions.html

My afternoon workshop offered the first, simplified version of the guided recitation included in this book. The next morning, I asked a palliative care doctor I'll call Zola about her experience of the 90-minute workshop. In that conversation and a follow-up email, Zola said that she lived in LA and had made her rounds that morning before returning to the conference. She reflected on a patient who was at that moment dying a very hard death. He was septic, with endstage comorbidities, and had just undergone a partial leg amputation. Gangrene had returned and the surgeons were recommending a second amputation. Zola said that prior to experiencing the Matrix, she would have counseled her patient-family on quality of life issues and the burden of suffering that would accompany additional efforts to forestall death—implicitly accepting additional amputations. The morning after experiencing the Matrix workshop she offered the afflicted man's wife something different. Zola voiced the reality that the husband was slowly dying, factually described what "doing everything" meant, and suggested how the couple's remaining time together would be if they let go of futile medical interventions prolonging death. Zola opened the possibility for this couple to choose a more peaceful way of dying, even given the advanced nature of their circumstances.

Zola's patient was dying at the endstage of medically managed diseases, under the control of medicine and perhaps even life-support machinery. By changing the way she counseled her patient's wife, Zola may have saved this couple from additional painful days or weeks in their end-of-life crucible. At the least, she honestly described the stark choices ahead of them.

As a result of her Matrix workshop participation, Zola's thousands of future patients will benefit from her more nuanced counsel. Windrum's Matrix of Dying Terms offers all of us—patients, family members, loved ones, and medical professionals alike—a new end-of-life tableau through which to aim for the types of deaths that most of us say we prefer, and away from the dying situations that we say we do not want to experience—situations that taken altogether I call our dying territory.

— —

I never thought to frame dying situations using terms like "delayed," suspended," "erroneous," "endstate," "collaborative," "abrupt," and "medically managed" until the fall of 2012 when seeds of Windrum's Matrix began germinating. Suspended dying and Erroneous dying are among the hardest dying situations to experience in our dying territory. It's one thing to vaguely say "I don't want to end up in the ICU; I want to die at home." It's another thing to distinctly foresee and consider all the end-of-life places we do end up—the range of dying situations where each and all of us land. To fully appreciate our need to foresee and plan, to really stimulate us to study up in advance, we need new language to identify and distinguish between our modern dying situations. My family didn't have it then. *The Promised Landing* introduces it now.

We were, family and medical people alike, doing the best we could, given our conditioning, limited knowledge and skill, and the prevailing precepts. Those precepts largely persist. Medicine delays and obfuscates because it doesn't perceive providing humane support for dying as part of its mission. Civilians deny that death will occur, refuse to look at it, and instead just hope that "things" will work out. What could possibly go wrong? Well, many things, for millions of dying people over generations' worth of time, with reverberating effect in the hearts of surviving loved ones.

Here is a simplified pictorial representation of our dying territory with the terms from the preceding stories placed within it: Delayed and Suspended dying for our experience of Mom's demise; Erroneous and Endstate dying for our experience of Dad's demise (including our brief traversal of Collaborative dying); and Endstate dying for what I presume Zola's patient and his wife experienced.

Understanding Demises as Destinations

Our Dying Territory

Controlling Forces ↓	Immediate		Time		Prolonged →
	Erroneous			Endstate	
		Delayed	Suspended		
			Collaborative		

These dying situations appear highlighted in the array below, a preview of the complete Matrix:

Windrum's Matrix of Dying Terms ™

Control	Abrupt Dying	Medically managed Dying			Never-ending Dying
		Onset	Progressed	Endstage	
World	Sudden	Insleep			SlowMotion
Medical	**Erroneous**	Early	Midstream	**Endstate**	
Machine	Emergency Room	**Delayed**	**Suspended**	Repetitive	Vegetative
Personal	Suicidal	Released	Postponed	Failed	
Shared		**Collaborative**			

LEGAL and/or ACCEPTED	ILLEGAL and/or UNACCEPTED	BOTH and/or AMBIGUOUS

At this point, it's not necessary that you try to divine the meaning of everything in Windrum's Matrix of Dying Terms. Fully understanding our dying territory, as the Matrix represents, requires extended explanation, and that's coming. First, we will explore our need of it. Next, the Glossary of Thoughts introduces key concepts that I use. Chapters 1–7 address each element step by step, sequentially revealing our dying territory. Chapter 8 offers vignettes that portray typical dying situations identified by each of the 17 terms. Chapter 9, the recitation, provides the opportunity for you to literally voice the possibility of experiencing each situation and gauge your visceral response to each. It will move your experience of this material out of your head and straight into your heart, gut, and soul. Chapter 10 zooms out, placing the Matrix in the context of the seven obstacles to dying in peace that comprise my end-of-life lexicon, To Die in Peace: Our Rights of Passage.

Throughout the years since my parents died, I've given much thought to why my family failed to find peaceful deaths and how each of us today can better aim for peaceful dying given the world we live in. The answers that have occurred to me seem valid, useful, and reliable—and widely overlooked, even as our society takes initial steps toward "death literacy." Accompany me through this book, and your understanding of modern dying will expand. You'll have new language with which to consider, discuss, and plan for your own and your loved ones' end days. A new perspective will emerge and serve as a baseline upon which you can increase your likelihood of experiencing the type of death we all say that we want for ourselves and for our loved ones, yet which remains elusive for too many of us.

Promises, Promises

For sentient beings here on planet Earth, dying may be painful enough in and of itself, and losing loved ones is existentially painful. Medicine has blessed us with beneficence over the past several generations, yet left unchecked, our medical system too often adds a second, unnecessary level of pain. Many families' experience of modern dying leaves bitterness about their experiences in the medical domain. The recent emergence of a social movement to relieve both levels of pain by learning how to prepare for and accept dying ironically adds the potential for a third level of pain.

The deaths I've experienced—my parents' sudden-onset, multi-week, error-filled hospitalized demises—revealed the distinction between *intrinsic* and *extrinsic* pain. Intrinsic pain is part of living and dying, plain and simple. Regarding the end of life, extrinsic pain is additional, unnecessary distress resulting from the nature and machinations of our technologically rich and relationship-poor medical system, abetted by our collective naiveté and willfully ignorant approach to dying. And now the likelihood looms for additional suffering emanating from unfulfilled promises.

The promises come from three sources. One source is medicine, through its wise guidance to execute advance directive documents and to assign a proxy to assist and/or represent us medically. (Advance directives are meant to specify what medical treatments people will allow and disallow. A proxy—also referred to as a surrogate or a healthcare agent—is a person authorized to act on our behalf, according to our instructions, when we cannot speak for ourselves.) Another source of promises is spiritual guidance intended to both calm us and reinforce our inner fortitude.

Although both are useful, each, I believe, implies that following the offered guidance will significantly increase our likelihood of dying peacefully rather than connected to unwanted life supports—a decidedly non-peaceful experience for many patient-families.

The third source of promises is us. Having collectively experienced millions of overmedicalized deaths, many of us, individually and collectively, are striving to become death-literate and death-accepting, promising ourselves "never again in my family or among my loved ones." We believe this promise will be fulfilled because we filled out legal directives and/or engaged in spiritual practice, certain that we have received enough information and knowledge to succeed.

We have not. And should these promises fail, whether they were implied from sources outside ourselves or emanating from within, and we end up landing in the types of dying situations we've vowed never to experience again, we add a new, third level of end-of-life pain: *promise pain*. Imagine for a long moment looking back on a loved one's demise in which all three levels of pain were part of your experience. As one who has experienced intrinsic and extrinsic end-of-life pain combined, I can tell you that I do not want promise pain added to future deaths in my family—nor to our memories. Nor to yours.

Why might we experience promise pain? My 14-year examination of end-of-life matters leads me to see clearly that practical education in identifying and learning how to mitigate obstacles to peaceful dying is crucially important—and virtually absent from civil and medical conversations. Given how medicalized, death-denying, and controlling our society is, I do not believe that directives and novice proxies and enriched spirit can, alone or together, act as a bulwark against inevitable and multiple obstacles to dying in peace.

Obstacles may develop slowly or arise instantaneously. They are linked, appearing simultaneously or in predictable sequence. They are persistent and shocking, ambushing us deep within our dying territory. We enter our dying realm with insufficient knowledge to plot our course through it, with no sense of impending obstacles and no map of its contours or way stations.

Our practical unpreparedness overwhelms the promise implied by directives, spiritual activation, and our own awakened longing.

I'm aware of a proliferation of offerings and enterprises to help people ponder, make, store, and access advance directives. I've read of many (and experienced several) spiritual teachings intended to enrich our inner selves, to instill both an open heart and a firm, if abstract, resolve. Yet I've seen no map of our dying territory with which to orient ourselves; no map naming well-known dying situations and showing their existence; no map with legends stimulating us to learn to identify, understand, and mitigate the range of everyday practical obstacles that await us throughout our dying territory.

The Promised Landing maps that territory. We will explore all its contours, ending our tour with a deepened appreciation of obstacles ahead and perhaps a resolve to learn what we must do, beyond directives and inner work, to overcome them so that we might increase our likelihood of dying *in* peace, and of dying *at* peace.

— —

I recall being locked out of my early childhood row house by Marta, whom my mother Ruth hired weekly for cleaning. Mom was a part-time bookkeeper; presumably Marta's duties included an hour or so of childcare after school that one day per week. Marta couldn't stand that I would tarnish the gleaming perfection she had made of Mom's kitchen, so she wouldn't let me in. I'd hover outside, six years old, skinny and bespectacled, hungry, wondering on what basis this other could lock me out of our home, awaiting some promised after-school care. Instead, Marta would unlock the door several minutes before Mom was due to arrive and threaten me to stay out of the kitchen.

We lived on Avenue X, low in the Sheepshead Bay neighborhood of Brooklyn, New York, a quintessential ethnic melting pot. Both my sets of grandparents were Lithuanian immigrants who spoke heavily accented English. Mom would occasionally get hooked by some turn of phrase, especially when it was delivered in one or another European accent. Later, after we'd moved to West Hempstead out on Long Island, she annoyed my fifth-grade teacher, Mr. Zungola, who took offense to a poem she'd written in "Italianesque." She had shared it with him thinking he'd appreciate its cleverness. Which brings me back to Marta who, in addition to locking the wee Bart out of his house, at some conversational point had said to Mom, "We grow too soon old and too late smart." In her middle and later years Mom would recite the proverb at moments when life seemed to get the better of one of us, pronouncing "oldt" and "schmaart" in Marta's German accent.

Perhaps the lockouts were the start of my distrust of authority. We lived in a naive age, an age that extends to the present for many when it comes to medical matters, especially the notion of being cared for near and at the end of life. Intelligent (but not yet smart) adult humans can and do wait for days on end during a loved one's medical emergencies, locked out of informed engagement, waiting for promised care. The medical system promises and trades on care although it doesn't define care the same way that civilians do and doesn't tell us so. We have to learn this ourselves, during poignant events, based both on what we do experience and what we do not experience. An important, perhaps crucial week may go by before we recognize that what's actually being delivered are medical treatments, sometimes care-fully, sometimes care-lessly, occasionally with care as families understand care. I learned this lesson in my early fifties, too "oldt" and too late to help my parents—but not too late to help others.

If I ever find Aladdin's magic lamp with its wish-granting genie, I'll ask to be smart. Smart would make me a quick and accurate assessor of situations in which I find myself. Smart would make me an immediately effective communicator. Smart would have made my sister and me instantly aware of the true nature of each of our family's 21st century hospitalizations instead of naively waiting for care, groping our way through demises that we had mistakenly thought our rule-abiding parents had planned well to avoid. Had we known of the obstacles to peaceful dying ahead of us, we might have become better equipped to avoid them.

Upon completing *The Promised Landing*, you will be much smarter when you find yourself in your moments of greatest need than I was when I found myself in mine. This is true for those who have already done end-of-life advance planning as well as for those who have not; for those who are spiritually engaged and for those who are not. You'll have a comprehensive map of our dying territory. You'll recognize the "lay of the land." You'll have sensitized yourself to the existence and nature of the full range of dying situations. You'll be able to sense or foresee what's on, or over, your horizon. You'll become a more rapid and accurate assessor of dying situations as they arise, and possibly before.

And as you continue learning about impediments to peaceful dying and how to manage them, you'll be better equipped to forecast and communicate your late-life and end-of-life wishes and to remain resolute regarding them. You'll become more confident, perhaps agile, in protecting yourself and your loved ones from entrapment in situations that you may say, or even vow, that you do not want to experience. You may even decide in advance to aim for dying situations that you'd prefer to experience. You'll be better equipped to fulfill your promises.

This larger, hopeful aspect of promise is the meaning I intend by the title *The Promised Landing: A Gateway to Peaceful Dying*. Herein is a new viewpoint and solution to a problem we've sensed but have literally lacked the language to broach, investigate, and articulate. Until now.

Glossary of Thoughts

In *The Promised Landing*, I make new distinctions—parsing and refining the use of existing words and introducing new language where none has previously been applied.

Throughout *The Promised Landing*, I refer to "dying in peace" and "dying at peace." Although I distinguish between these, they combine to form a unified experience that unfolds over time and culminates in a moment. That process (one's demise) and that moment (death) form a continuum, shared equally by dying persons and their attending loved ones (the "patient-family"). When discussing these matters, I always have the patient-family experience in mind.

By "peace" I mean the absence of strife or shock and the harm that results from experiencing either, which is usually heightened due to the patient-family's vulnerability during a loved one's demise.

Although "demise" and "death" are dictionary synonyms, I use "demise" to refer to the months, weeks, and days of decline, and "death" to refer to the moment when we die.

"Situation" and "circumstances" are dictionary synonyms that I distinguish between, with the former encompassing and made up of the latter. A situation is the scene; circumstances are the myriad details brought by all involved to that scene. Our focus herein is not on circumstances—for example, any particular disease or cause of death, or our personalities; our focus is on our experience of dying at the convergence of some point in the progression of a demise and whatever predominantly controls the situation. We bring our circumstances to some situation (which also contains its own circumstances) and we take them away with us when we leave.

Within this book I use the words "surrogate," "proxy," and "healthcare agent" to refer to people we designate through legal documents to represent and enforce our wishes about medical matters when we are unable to speak for ourselves. In some jurisdictions, "proxy" has another specific legal meaning; that is not my intent in this discussion.

By "engage medically" I mean to seek, undergo, or acquiesce to medical tests or treatments, generally of the more invasive or risky kind (risk is a moving target affected by age, condition, treatments, and environments).

The Promised Landing introduces Windrum's Matrix of Dying Terms as a lens through which to more clearly understand the implications of our choices. "Matrix" may seem like an unusual term. I use it to describe the full range of dying situations, each of which is distinctly different in our experience. Its several definitions are particularly meaningful for people seeking peace near and at the end of life:

• A matrix is an environment in which something develops—as anyone involved in protracted dying situations deeply experiences.

• A matrix is also a mold in which something is cast—those involved in late-life situations where inexplicable forces commingle come to feel emotionally molded by them, sometimes permanently.

• And a matrix is an array of mathematical expressions (a simple expression is the equation $2+2=4$ where the 2s are symbols, the = is an operator, and 4 is the value). Just as a mathematical matrix displays values arrayed across a table, Windrum's Matrix depicts our dying situations arrayed across our dying territory—a place where we'd like things to "add up" and for our experiences to reflect our values.

This small word, matrix, packs a lot of meaning. *The Promised Landing* unpacks a unique end-of-life Matrix and in so doing, offers a gateway to peaceful dying.

Impetus

This book is a direct result of unanimous feedback I received from a dozen participants in a March 2015 focus group in which I summarized "To Die in Peace: Your Rights of Passage." That program identifies and unravels a series of obstacles that we must mitigate or, even better, overcome in order to increase our likelihood of dying in peace. I identify 10 obstacles. For three that lay outside the lexicon—beliefs, family relations, and financial wherewithal—I have no guidance, for these vexing matters are deeply personal. Of the other seven I have a great deal to say—I have experienced them more than once (see chapter 10 for that discussion).

My solution to one obstacle in particular—difficulty distinguishing among dying situations—captured the group's attention. *The Promised Landing* focuses on it. *Failure to distinguish between distinctly different dying situations means that we are unlikely to anticipate them.* And so we get stuck in situations that add extrinsic and even promise pain to the pain that's intrinsic to dying and loss.

Lacking names for these situations, lacking the language with which to discuss them, is a chicken-and-egg scenario: do we fail to distinguish because we lack the language, or do we lack the language because we fail to distinguish? In either case, the solution is to consider what shapes our dying time in general and our dying experiences more specifically. And then to formulate names by which we may distinguish between the full range of dying situations in our modern world. We can see and understand our dying time as a territory we must traverse, with way stations and destinations that we can identify by their core characteristics. Each situation is named according to its essential nature, that is, *our experience of it*.

We've been oversimplifying matters by describing only several scenes—the feared worst: attached to life-support machinery in a hospital ICU where we understand little and control less; the rosy best: independently at home, lovingly and adequately cared for, the family pet at hand, free to make the non-medical as important as the medical; and our communal nightmare: demented years in abusive nursing homes.

The focus group members, long-tenured end-of-life professionals (nurses, chaplains, educators) and deeply experienced laypeople who had, like me, become end-of-life reform activists, unanimously said that the solution of naming dying situations was the first thing I should present to everybody, both civilians and medical professionals; that this was a gateway to all the end-of-life guidance I offer.

Let's take a tour through our dying territory, learning to see it anew through the lens of Windrum's Matrix of Dying Terms.

Our Dying Territory:
Identifying and Naming Our Dying Situations
Windrum's Matrix of Dying Terms

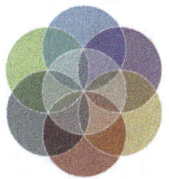

Chapter 1

Matrix Underpinnings: Promises and Practicalities

Why do we need more words for dying? Because we have lacked the language to articulate what dying has become for us. Because we cannot adequately describe our reality. Because dying in peace and at peace require that we have an unambiguous view of what lies ahead. Because implied promises lull us into unpreparedness. Because fulfilling end-of-life promises requires a healthy dose of the practical.

A promise is a declaration or assurance that a particular thing will happen. Especially regarding the end of life, promises raise hope and create expectations. My perspective is that much of what's offered today as guidance for achieving "a good death" implies that following that guidance is enough to ensure a peaceful demise. Guidance regarding end-of-life matters comes mainly from medicine and spiritual practitioners. Medicine encourages—even exhorts—us to have those challenging conversations about dying and death with our loved ones; to fill out at least one or even several legal forms (collectively referred to as advance directives); and to assign a surrogate to ensure our wishes are met should we become unable to manage for ourselves. As a graphic designer, I've laid out and formatted some of these informative materials myself, and over the years I've seen several iterations of both the forms and social movements proposing one or another approach to the hard work of preparing oneself to complete them.

Even more nuanced issues and advance directive documents exist beyond the basic three (Living Will, medical durable power of attorney, and some flavor of resuscitation directive; see Appendix C for more), and we are all well-advised to fill out and have on hand directives that may apply to us. Medical guidance seems to suggest—or the public seems to believe—that showing up with documents in hand and an untested surrogate beside us, months or years after drafting directives, during what is likely to be an existential medical crisis, will ensure that a demise is peaceful for the dying and their loved ones. This is a misleading implication at best and a false promise at worst.

Spiritual practitioners, including the secular spiritual eldering movement, offer an array of trainings and workshops related to death acceptance. Some include rituals. The several I've experienced induce a softening of heart as an antidote to emotional paralysis and the fear expressed in our cultural denial of death. Buddhism is infused with rigorous practices to help us accept impermanence and balance desire with the deeper truths of existence.

Having experienced too many overmedicalized deaths of loved ones, people today are becoming more desirous of peaceful dying. Growing numbers are attending discussion events such as Death Cafes, exploring advance directives through organizations such as The Conversation Project, as well as engaging in some sort of spiritual practice.

These pursuits are valid, useful, and necessary. Missing is the third leg of an end-of-life management tripod: examination of the everyday practical obstacles that our social-medical-corporate-legal system places in our way. There are many. They are severe. They are unexpected. They arise quickly. They have persisted for generations and any combination of obstacles is likely to pop up within any given demise, despite any implied promises from any source. Taken together, these obstacles are what I refer to as "systemic defaults." Medicine typically does not broach their existence, and we remain uneducated about them—until we're in the middle of a demise going from bad to worse.

That we so want a peaceful death makes plainly evident how sacred our dying time is for each of us—and for our loved ones. And how elusive dying in and at peace has become for most of us. Although we might luck out and die without strife, doing nothing other than taking a final breath, today's world is so undersupportive and overcontrolling and dying is so overmedicalized, that assuming we will just luck our way out is foolish at best.

When asked, most of us will say, "I want to die in peace." I believe that we misconstrue that small word "in," referring to how we want to feel and be at the moment we die. A better way to express that desire is, "I want to die *at* peace." Experiencing my parents' deaths taught me that we're not likely to die at peace if the experiences leading to our deaths are not peaceful. Dying *in* peace refers to those experiences over the months, weeks, and days of our demise. I express this distinction in the first line of the Never Say Die Rap, intoning "Want to die AT peace? Got to die IN peace."

A range of shortcomings exists with traditional end-of-life preparatory guidance. Assigning a proxy is a starting point, but learning how to advocate for ourselves or for our loved ones as that proxy is daunting. It's a time-consuming endeavor requiring self-directed study to find guidance (most of the best is offered by laypeople who share what they have learned through painful experience). Medicine doesn't discuss this with us because deeply learning in advance what we need to know to function as medical proxies would reveal pitfalls of our medical system that the system would prefer remain unpublicized. And most people wouldn't even believe such possibilities until they experience them—at which point we're in one of those situations we'd previously vowed to avoid, and which are infamously hard, even impossible, to extricate ourselves from.

Spiritual engagement offers the potential to develop two important personal character traits: equanimity and resolve. Equanimity, or composure under pressure, is of great benefit and even necessary in medical situations, especially life and death. If you're like me, equanimity doesn't come naturally; it must be learned (and re-learned) and consciously called upon. Resolve is necessary to stay one's course. We must manifest great resolve should our preferences run counter to pressures exerted by the medical system to accept more medical treatment than we desire. This is especially true in situations in which we are at a disadvantage—possessing less technical medical knowledge and feeling less powerful than medical professionals, and perhaps subject to conflicting pressures from doctors, family members, friends, or even our community.

How do we apply equanimity and resolve as developed in the loving quietude of spiritual practice when we are suddenly enmeshed in red-alert circumstances, or over time in order to try to steer clear of such situations? The key is learning exactly what those situations are made of, in advance, so that we may recognize and anticipate them. Medical matters generally, and life-and-death matters specifically, are subject to many internal and external forces about which we have vague inklings but rarely have prior or deep experience. Since we don't learn about them in advance (that's death denial in action or better put, death-denial *in*action), I suggest that learning equanimity and resolve without also learning about ever-present obstacles to dying in peace leaves us at full risk of enduring experiences that we say we want to avoid—and of surviving loved ones living thereafter with those technicolor memories.

We aspire to die in peace, but we don't know how to overcome today's many impediments because we haven't identified or considered them. Our aspiration for peaceful deaths results in promises—be they implied, expressed, or merely hoped for. The promise we want fulfilled is to land gently when our music stops. To literally come to Earth in peace. Most of us will require learned skills in order to orient ourselves toward the landing we want and, as importantly, away from the landings we don't want. In my experience and in my end-of-life lexicon, our ability to keep our own promises requires significant prior study and understanding to learn about practicalities that are, especially on first exposure, disheartening. Doing so starts with unambiguous analysis and assessment, which requires clear, non-euphemistic language. Our actions are based on our thoughts, and if we haven't thought through our dying territory, we simply do not know how to act or where to turn once we, or a loved one, enters it. Let's enter it now, assess its contours, and identify its way stations.

Chapter 2

Matrix Genesis: A Zillion Words for Snow

It's not that words fail us; it's that the absence of words fails us...

I began working on end-of-life matters in 2004 and had been developing and presenting guidance for dying in peace for eight years. One day during fall 2012, I arose from my garden level basement workspace to stretch my legs and relax my mind. My office occupies one quadrant of the space. My sit-to-stand computer table and a cabinet topped with bindery equipment serve as a room divider. That afternoon, standing in the "theater zone" between a love seat, recliners, and white marble Saarinen table, a thought unrelated to anything in particular popped unbidden into my head:

*Eskimos have a zillion words for snow.
How come we have only one word for dying?*

This thought stopped me in my tracks. The refined question would be, "The Inuit have many words for snow. Why have we Anglos only one non-euphemistic word for dying?" but that's not how the thought arrived. Regardless, let's examine its parts. A zillion of course is exaggerated, but northern peoples do have many words to describe snow in its various forms. This cliché observation is paired with the implication that English has an inadequate range of expressions for snow in particular, and, perhaps a similar deficit for other aspects of life, too. Actually we do have some number of snow words: crust, flurries, powder, sleet, slush, spindrift, whiteout. Skiers have numerous additional descriptors: boilerplate, champagne, corduroy, corn, crud, death cookies, dust, fluff, graupel, junk, mashed potatoes, peanut butter, set-up, wet cement. We're obviously not bereft of an ability to analyze our experiences and express distinctions.

We haven't, in large part, applied these skills to end-of-life language except to hide. We have but one word to describe our experience of dying: "dying"—except for euphemisms. Here are some I find most evocative: Bite the dust. Buy the farm. Cash in your chips. Check out. Croak. Cross over. Depart. Give up the ghost. Go to your reward. Kick the bucket. Meet your maker. Shuffle off this mortal coil. Pushing up daisies.

These clever expressions allow us to hide from death, especially from how we experience dying in the late 20th and early 21st centuries. None of these descriptions convey anything about the nature of our experiences during the months, weeks, and days of a demise or the moment of death. Nor what our society has made of late life and dying.

This no-words-for-dying notion stole my attention. I couldn't un-think it. The construct sat like a skullcap. I sensed depth within it. My quest as "a grain of sand in the end-of-life oyster" (or less colorfully put, a lay person turned end-of-life reform advocate) has its roots in language. I rely upon identifying words and concepts that describe the nature of our dying experiences. I'd spent a decade unraveling end-of-life complexities and suddenly, this thought…

Eskimos have a zillion words for snow.
How come we have only one word for dying?

When we envision dying, usually a trio of disparate situations come to mind. Many of us say, "I don't want to end up wired up in the ICU," by which we mean attached to intravenous lines, perhaps an airway ventilator, even a feeding tube, surrounded by a phalanx of machine readouts and doctors and nurses taking marching orders from them. In response to this now-classic scene, others say, "I want to die at home," supposedly a pastoral setting with familiar walls, pets, friends, and reliable caregivers offering uninterrupted medical and social comforts and lovingkindness. Finally, we remember to add the specter of dwindling for years in a nursing facility.

What we're describing when envisioning these outcomes are *scenes*. We see these tableaux and imagine ourselves as the principal actor within them. These binary scenes seem to be all we ever imagine. ICU or nursing home; nursing home or our own home. As if no other dying episodes exist, regardless of numerous and prevalent factors that influence, shape, or control our demises.

In fact, a range of dying *situations* lies in front of us. The dictionary defines a situation as a "state of affairs" and lists "circumstances" as a synonym. I prefer more precise distinctions when discussing end-of-life matters. In my view, circumstances are the myriad details of our lives. Dying situations are made of many circumstances… our particular ailments or diseases, temperaments and (in)tolerances, family relations, finances, histories, and so on. Add in the personalities and systems that make up the non-us part of the situation—for example, the "medical system" with its never-say-die default orientation and government regulations that shape medical practice. Together, all the circumstances become a situation in which we could find ourselves. Situations that we collectively imagine, that are part of our zeitgeist, have become ingrained in our psyches as scenes. And a corollary: *situations for which we have no names do not enter our psyche at all. Nor do they enter our thinking, our conversations, and certainly not our planning and resolve.*

Why must we resolve so assiduously? What must we plan for so steadfastly in order to increase our likelihood of dying in peace? It's not that we're all at risk of being attacked by bears, dragged off by alligators, chomped on by sharks; comparatively few of us die in vehicle wrecks; fewer in industrial accidents or natural disasters; and although the numbers by themselves are staggering, only a fraction of us in the United States die by gunfire. What is all this planning and resolving meant to protect us from?

Ourselves. The system we've created. Our strange culture of dying and death that's evolved over many generations—the reasons for which lay beyond this book's focus yet are responsible for this work's existence.

> *Eskimos have a zillion words for snow.*
> *How come we have only one word for dying?*

I called a friend and colleague, a whip-smart academic, end-of-life policy analyst, and end-of-life ethicist who knew what was and wasn't happening in the palliative care and hospice worlds. I asked if anyone locally, regionally, or nationally (USA) had examined the question and published about it. The answer, simply, was no.

A brief complimentary search of academic articles conducted for me at the University of Colorado Anschutz Medical School library indicated that when language was a focus of publications addressing death and dying, those works delved into psychology.*

I decided to answer the unbidden question myself. The fact that I didn't consciously ask, or ask for, the question became a demand for my complete attention. The result, after three months' time,

---

*The librarian ran a search of three academic journal databases: PsychINFO, EBSCO Psych and Behavioral Sciences, and Ovid Medline (PubMed), bringing back the first 100 citations from each source on a search of the following parameters:
1. (death or dead or dying).ti. or exp "death and dying"/ or exp death anxiety/ or exp death attitudes/ or exp death education/ or death rites/
2. (Semantic* or syntax or communication* or metaphor* or language* or euphemism* or metonym* or allegor* or symbol* or narration).tw. or exp language/ or exp rhetoric/ or exp symbolism/ or exp verbal communication/
3. 1 and 2

The search did not include so-called gray literature—nonpublished conference abstracts and proceedings, writings from think tanks, and other materials that don't appear in academic journals; popular culture; nor MBase (the European equivalent of PubMed).

was Windrum's Matrix of Dying Terms. I wound up devoting almost one-third of my 2013 TEDxFoCo talk to it ("Dying IN Peace to Die AT Peace: New Terms of Engagement," viewable at AxiomAction.com/speaking). While re-watching the recording recently, I heard myself introduce the Matrix by saying "I think that if we overcome this obstacle, it will help us anticipate and overcome all the others." It was an accidental statement uttered in response to realizing that as I performed the "Never Say Die Rap," my Rap slide had advanced to a Matrix slide as the controller got squeezed in my jacket pocket. Writing this now, I smile, amused that two years later a focus group unanimously reminded me that this was their assessment, too.

Chapter 3

Matrix Basics: Cardinal Aspects

Imagine if our planet's hundreds of thousands of unique flowers had no names. Not a one. And that the only word we had to refer to any and all of them was "flower."

How would we distinguish between them? How could we state our preferences? How would we specify bouquets?

Without names for obviously different flowers, the answer to these questions would be "with great difficulty and with limited, if any, success." Actually, it's hard to imagine a world in which all the flowers we appreciate went unnamed. Or, for that matter, numerous other sets which represent different instances of things such as spices, dog breeds, musical artists, software properties, chemical elements, family members, friends, colleagues…

This sole word, "dying," fails to describe the destinations within our dying territory or even convey that there are any. Using only this word limits our ability, privately in our thoughts and together in conversation, to distinguish among different dying experiences.

As with flowers, dying situations differ from each other. Different situations are different experiences. Granted, it's easier to observe differences between objects than situations, especially if we haven't already lived through some. But don't you have a gnawing sense that the cliché binary choice of dying either in an ICU or at home doesn't quite describe the full range of final scenes we might inhabit? We've all heard stories, some within our own families, of end-of-life scenarios that were needlessly rough on the dying and left survivors distraught. Over generations and many years, we've accumulated too many such stories. Our future scenes are predictable because they have proven, unfortunately, to be real. We just haven't formally identified and named them.

Time

If "dying" encompasses a set of situations, how do we begin to discern what they're made of? This was the first question I needed to answer. To do it I asked, "What are the elemental aspects of dying that shape our experience of it?" I identified two cardinal aspects: time and control. Having two parameters suggested that I represent our dying territory with a table. Simple two-dimensional tables have two axes, vertical and horizontal. It seemed apt to place Time on the horizontal axis:

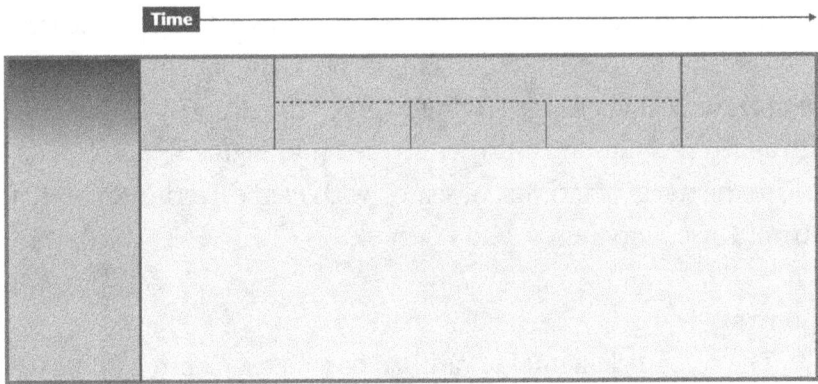

We approach our dying time, or a loved one's, in one of two ways, or even both sequentially depending on how long the dying time extends. If one wants to live, one asks "How much time do I have?" If one wants dying to end, one asks "How long is this going to take?" Windrum's Matrix divides time into three primary durations with the middle duration further divided into three. I used medical terms for the evolution of disease to name the middle durations:

	Immediate ——————————— Time ——————————— Prolonged →			
Abrupt Dying	**Medically managed Dying**			**Never-ending Dying**
	Onset	Progressed	Endstage	

The three primary timeframes are Abrupt, Medically managed, and Never-ending. Abrupt dying refers to deaths that occur instantaneously or from a particular cause that irreversibly supersedes other trajectories, an aspect that I'll explain further on. Never-ending dying refers to drawn-out demises that place dying people (and their attending loved ones) in a queer place unique to our modern world. Medically managed dying refers to the majority of deaths in advanced societies. It is further divided into segments corresponding to the stages of terminal diseases, with medical terms to identify them: Onset, Progressed, and Endstage.

Control

The second elemental or cardinal parameter, Control, populates the vertical axis:

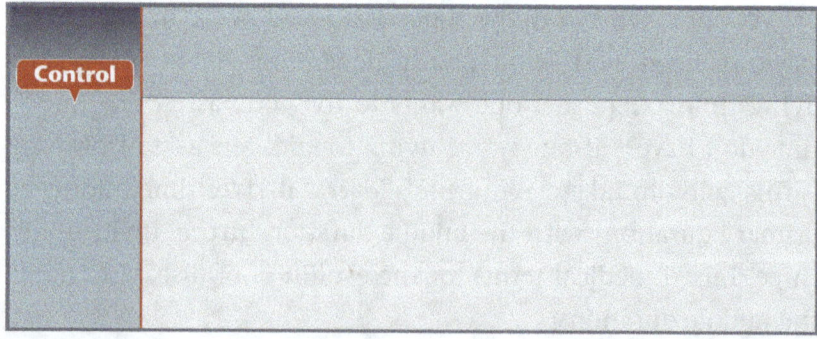

Five controls identify what or who might exert predominant control over our dying experience: the World, Medicine, Machines, Personal, and Shared, exemplified below with badges:

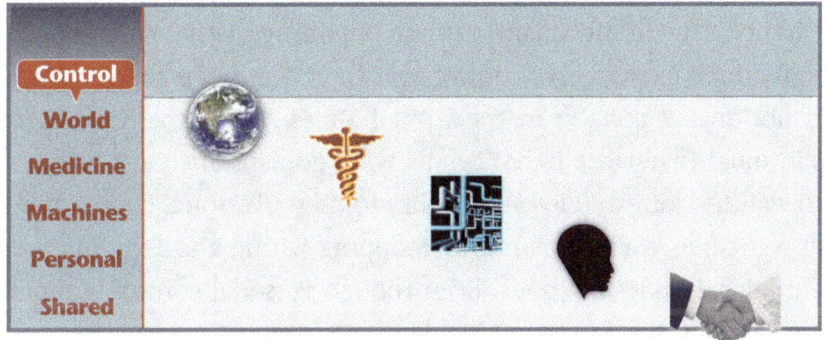

Controls have certain characteristics:

When the World has control over dying, we have none; something completely beyond our agency causes death to occur.

Medical control shapes the majority of deaths today. Most deaths occur within institutions. And we all embrace medicine's beneficence, wherever we are, because it is so effective; even at-home deaths will be medicalized. Medical control offers some advantages: it can be provided across multiple settings and delivery can be modified to fit changing health circumstances or patient-proxy desires. In other words, medical control offers, to some degree, flexibility and mobility.

Machine control refers to life-support equipment and methods: ventilator (breathing machine) intubation, central lines into airways and gut, and intensive machine monitoring. Once "hooked up," one is immobilized in that setting. And once these interventions are installed, it can be extremely hard to reverse course and remove them—much more so than many people believe it ethically ought to be. Machine control also applies to implanted medical life-support devices (which the bearers have the ethical right to have deactivated; that right has been made legal in some jurisdictions, yet deactivation may have to be fought for.).

Personal control refers to shaping the timing and nature of one's own death, what I term "self-directed dying." Three pathways exist. The first is Medical Aid in Dying (MAID), also known as Physician Assisted Dying and by the popular phrase Death With Dignity. After legally qualifying and obtaining a lethal prescription, individuals exercise sole control over their deaths. Personal control is not always certain; in the United States, where the dying person must ingest the lethal agents with no assistance, it's possible to wait too long and lose the ability to do so. Personal control may also include VSED (Voluntarily Stopping Eating and Drinking) or extra-legal "exit" methods. Even though Personal control is about enablement, the specter of disablement grows as time passes.

Shared control refers to engaging hospice services well in advance of life's final days, known as active dying, with ample time for families to be assisted with managing a loved one's demise and death. Our experience with hospice will depend upon a range of variables because hospice organizations range in organization, size and resources, and service offerings. Shared control should confer greater ease and peace, although the potential for tension is present due to differing capabilities of different hospice agencies.

— —

So here we are, knowing that our demises unfold over time—time during which we are very much alive. Predominantly, complex systems outside of ourselves exert fundamental control over our end days and our dying situations, and their values may differ from ours. At this point, our dying territory is an undifferentiated, extensive space:

MATRIX BASICS

	Abrupt Dying	Medically managed Dying			Never-ending Dying
Control		Onset	Progressed	Endstage	
World					
Medical					
Machine					
Personal					
Shared					

Before populating the Matrix with place names, let us fly some banners over the space to remind ourselves again of our primary goal to die in peace and to acknowledge a goal for those who may desire extended life supports, each of which suggests why distinguishing among dying situations matters. Where across our dying territory must we land to attain these goals?

	Abrupt Dying	Medically managed Dying			Never-ending Dying
Control		Onset	Progressed	Endstage	
World					
Medical			**Peace**		
Machine					
Personal					
Shared					

	Abrupt Dying	Medically managed Dying			Never-ending Dying
Control		Onset	Progressed	Endstage	
World					
Medical			**Desire**		
Machine					
Personal					
Shared					

Chapter 4

Matrix Territory: Where're You Gonna Land?

The idea of landing somewhere is so common that we express it as an aphorism: "Landed in hot water" and "Where're you gonna land?"

Where are you going to land? indeed…. As with musical chairs: When the music stops, where're you gonna land? Or, akin to game boards, where pieces representing us move from square to square: When the game's over, where're you gonna land? In a place you've aimed for or a place you've stumbled into with no advance reconnoitering? In all seriousness, when our life game is over, in which dying situations would we prefer to land? In a situation we've actively planned to experience, or in a situation we wish we had never slipped into or become entrapped in?

"Landings" are spaces arrayed across Windrum's Matrix that represent distinctly different dying situations. Each landing represents the intersection, or combination, or mashup of who or what exerts predominant control and how long into a demise we enter active dying (life's final brief period) and experience our death.

Our Dying Territory: Landings

Control	Abrupt Dying	Medically managed Dying			Never-ending Dying
		Onset	Progressed	Endstage	
World					
Medical					
Machine					
Personal					
Shared					

So: We land in situations where our time runs out under the control of some entity, either abruptly, or sometime along a disease's course (or trajectory in medical parlance), or dragged out at some length.

Think of landings as destinations that appear on maps like towns, cities, mountaintops, and points of interest. Maps show us how we may travel through some region. Destinations are places we stop. At the end of life, we stop somewhere for good. And we get there by traversing, over time, our dying territory.

Control	Abrupt Dying	Medically managed Dying			Never-ending Dying
		Onset	Progressed	Endstage	
World					
Medical					
Machine					
Personal					
Shared					

Without knowing one thing more about this construct—a model of our everyday world—without yet naming any landing, perhaps you have the sense that you might prefer to land in certain places and not land in other places…

Chapter 5

Matrix Time-out: Metaphors and Billboards, Borders and Silos, Preferences, Neutrality, Duration

Before proceeding with our dying territory tour and naming Matrix landings, let's pause and reflect.

The Matrix is an end-of-life tool that is built on, and presents, precise thinking and wording to aid us in seeing what we sense awaits us but haven't yet named. As a model, it can both clarify and mislead. It offers insights, yet its structure with lines and boxes may suggest that it portrays a world that's simple and rigid, whereas our lives are more complex and fluid.

Metaphors and Billboards

To introduce a new concept for which we have yet to devise language, I have employed analogy—flowers with no names, and metaphor—a game board with spaces we land on "for good," as we say in English, along with road maps to suggest traversability. Graphically, I've used the space within the Matrix, soon to display landing names, as a sort of billboard, representing aspects of our dying territory by placing badges, peace and desire banners, a tiled game board, and a roadmap across its surface. Through these images, I introduce a vision of dying as a territory that we move through over time: a territory populated with way stations and destinations. A territory in which we have profound experiences during our final time on planet Earth.

The graphics I show within the Matrix when introducing its concepts are not the Matrix itself. The fallen traffic cones on the roadmap billboard convey a sense of rough roads and danger, and that's an editorial reflection. Rough times are intrinsic to dying at the end stages of terminal illnesses. Some people like the challenge of rough roads and find value in persevering through difficult times. The Matrix, as you will notice after we populate it with landing names, does not editorialize about what any person makes of rough times, of harder landings, or of softer ones. Some people will aim for landings that other people will vow to avoid; this applies in both directions—toward harder landings and toward softer landings.

Notice I wrote "aim for," not "choose" or "select." With few exceptions, neither I nor you can declare that we will die in this manner or that, at this time or that, in one situation or another. That's why I strive to speak and write in terms of "increasing or decreasing our likelihood" of experiencing one or another situation.

Porous Borders, No Silos

As with any journey, we may not simply go from point A to point Z; we may pass through way stations, or linger, or retrace our steps along the way. The Matrix—as the game board metaphor suggests—accommodates this. Because of time. And because we do have some agency to move toward or away from this or that controlling entity.

Windrum's Matrix of Dying Terms is a model. The layout's hard straight lines imply non-crossable boundaries. They imply that each landing is a world unto itself. That we'd have some serious fence climbing to do to move from one to another. That landings are silos, self-contained and filled with one thing only. They are none of this; landings are way stations throughout our dying territory. We make choices when traveling; we ponder and select routes and destinations. And then we set off, perhaps encountering unexpected closed roads and detours—obstacles, for purposes of this discussion.

Preferences

One aspect of life that the Matrix doesn't convey is preference. The Matrix has no preferences and doesn't account for mine or yours. That's what *we* bring to the model. What the Matrix stirs in us is a dawning awareness that:

- Our dying territory is made of situations that can be identified and named;
- Naming situations that differ from each other may help us clarify our preferences;
- Clarifying our preferences may stimulate us to learn how to modify our glide path in order to die in the manner we say we want.

Neutrality

It took me three months to complete the first full iteration of Windrum's Matrix, with most of that time spent seeking a set of neutral names for the landings. I explored sets of words that I felt emanated from practical considerations, emotional considerations, experiential considerations, and existential considerations. I finally realized that the Matrix required simple descriptors with no judgment about medicine or society or ourselves, and with no emotional charge. I was seeking single-word terms to accurately describe the essential nature of dying at a certain point in time, under the control of some predominant entity. I sought terms specific to each landing *situation* but not so overly specific as to function as commentary on some *circumstance*.

Duration

Landings do not relate to fixed durations; diseases develop and lives flow and ebb at different rates. The Matrix doesn't predict how much or how little time any of us may spend in any landing.

— —

Next, we'll see and interact with the landing names. First, we'll learn the 17 names. Then we'll describe each landing through vignettes typifying dying trajectories that would land us there. After that, we'll engage in a guided recitation to get out of our heads and experience the Matrix through our hearts, guts, and souls, trying each landing on for size.

Chapter 6

Matrix: Landings

Control	Abrupt Dying	Medically managed Dying			Never-ending Dying
		Onset	Progressed	Endstage	
World					
Medical					
Machine					
Personal					
Shared					

Windrum's Matrix of Dying Terms contains 17 landings with unique names representing distinctly different dying situations. We experience all of them collectively in our societies and one by one as individuals and patient-families.

You need not memorize their names. I haven't; ask me on any given day and I may have trouble naming more than several. But I never forget the depiction of our dying territory that Windrum's Matrix expresses.

Rote memorization is not the point. The Matrix is a tool, not a chore. We store tools when not in use and retrieve them when we need them. When we lack the right tool for some job, we fudge it. Or kludge. These words mean "to tinker" and "to use ill-assorted parts." We do what we can with what we have on hand. Fudging and kludging about end-of-life matters can land us in euphemistic hot water. When we want to make lasting repairs, we seek tools designed to do the job and learn how to use them. The 17 landing names, taken together, are such a tool. They help us do a job that we, individually and as a society, have needed help doing for a very long time. Matrix names capture and succinctly express the essential nature of our experience when we or a loved one dies in these situations. The Matrix helps us realize in concrete terms that dying situations differ from one another, and it suggests how.

When you need to refresh yourself about end-of-life matters, when late-life issues arise and require planning or enactment of a plan or changing the plan, remember this end-of-life tool called Windrum's Matrix of Dying Terms, reach for this book, review it, and (re)incorporate its meaning into your life. If you look for and find the Matrix through an online search, be sure any online image you refer to is gray-blue and contains 17 landings; the original published Matrix was predominantly bright green, with 16 landings (see Appendix D).

Becoming comfortable with 17 possibilities, memorized or not, is probably not as hard as you may initially think, for when you're engaged in a pursuit, you learn its building blocks. I propose that you can name, easily or with just a little effort, 17 items found within one or more sets of things that make up your life. Seventeen family members, friends, or colleagues? Rattle 'em off! Are you a landscaper? Seventeen flowers. Do you cook? Seventeen spices. Code software? Seventeen properties. A chemist? Seventeen elements. Car buff? Seventeen models. Love music? Seventeen songs. Study cinema? Seventeen flicks. Want to die in peace? Seventeen landings.

— —

A note about what landing names are not: landing names are not medical, technical, or scientific. They are not intended to be emotional triggers. They do not cast judgment, nor do they attempt to nudge us one way or another. They neither editorialize nor play favorites. Dying situation landing names do one thing: describe the essential nature of *the patient-family's experience* of active dying and death within a timeframe and under some predominant entity's control. "Within a timeframe" can imply that the patient-family has already traversed other landings, other way stations throughout our dying territory, although this may not be true in all cases. Landing names exist for one reason: to help us understand and envision distinctly different dying situations well in advance of experiencing them. This reason has a clear purpose: to help us decide if we'd be OK, or not OK, with experiencing certain landings, and to stimulate us to learn how to aim for those landings we are willing to experience and away from landings we are not willing to experience. For medical professionals, Windrum's Matrix's additional purpose is to serve as a stimulus to help you help patient-families through their end-of-life journey.

I have a favorite phrase to describe all this: New Terms of Engagement. "Terms" refers to words as identifiers as well as to conditions or understandings.

Now, let's identify the 17 landings that together make up our dying territory.

Insleep dying
throughout the Medically managed timeframe
under World control

Control	Abrupt Dying	Medically managed Dying			Never-ending Dying
		Onset	Progressed	Endstage	
World		Insleep			
Medical					
Machine					
Personal					
Shared					

Insleep dying may be the Holy Grail of dying situations; so many people cite dying in their sleep as their preferred landing. Insleep dying may be the least frightening way to go. Because it's non-threatening, we begin our dying territory tour on this landing. Insleep dying could occur within any landing. But that's not how we mean it when we express a preference to die in our sleep; we mean that we'd like to go easily, naturally, with no pain or drama, without extended medical engagement. It's likely that, for most people who die in their sleep, some amount of late-life medical management for one or more comorbidities has been part of their lives.

Sudden dying
within the Abrupt timeframe
under World control

Control	Abrupt Dying	Medically managed Dying			Never-ending Dying
		Onset	Progressed	Endstage	
World	Sudden	Insleep			
Medical					
Machine					
Personal					
Shared					

Sudden dying under World control refers to any type of natural disaster, a civic infrastructure failure, an accident, or death by violent means. Although we might try to avoid these events, there's nothing we can do about any of this landing's circumstances—the World controls.

Erroneous dying
within the Abrupt timeframe
under Medical control

Control	Abrupt Dying	Medically managed Dying			Never-ending Dying
		Onset	Progressed	Endstage	
World	Sudden		Insleep		
Medical	Erroneous				
Machine					
Personal					
Shared					

Errors in judgement regarding the advisability of undergoing one or another medical procedure, and medical error, alone or combined, can land us in Erroneous dying.

A precipitous change of trajectory may result from errors in judgement. When we hope for too much, when risks are undisclosed, unexamined, or unheeded, we expose ourselves to the potential for the very thing we wish to avoid. I examine what we might do to moderate this tendency when discussing one prevalent obstacle to peaceful dying, Trouble Determining When Enough is Enough (see chapter 10, Obstacles to Peaceful Dying and How to Mitigate Them).

Preventable medical error is the third leading cause of death in America. If you haven't already heard about this it's because the statistic is not well-publicized—neither directly tracked and correlated with death certificates, nor widely admitted to by medicine, nor much reported on. However, reliable government and industry studies issued in 1999, 2003, and 2010 have confirmed the prevalence of fatal preventable medical error.* Former U.S. Vice-President Joe Biden has spoken publicly and directly about this.**

I have contributed an article suggesting that *It's Time to Account for Medical Error in "Top Ten Causes of Death" Charts* (search for

"Windrum JoPM" to obtain the link or enter https://Participatory Medicine.org/journal/opinion/commentary/2013/04/24/it's-time-to-account-for-medical-error-in-"top-ten-causes-of-death-charts/).

As with errors of judgement, should preventable error occur as the causal factor leading to death, despite the presence of comorbidities, error has abruptly changed one's end-of-life trajectory. Its precipitous aspect qualifies Erroneous dying for placement within the Abrupt timeframe. Even if one's demise and death are not sudden, the introduction of error, the altered medical trajectory, and the debilitating destabilization of the patient-family are sudden and cataclysmic, especially if the error is medical.

Unless death occurs at the same time as a medical error, the patient-family will eventually land in some other Matrix landing. I categorize deaths instigated by medical error, regardless of any existing comorbidities, as Erroneous.

My family experienced Erroneous dying. We made errors in judgement, and late-life modern medicine failed us—either directly through its practice or due to the conditions under which such treatments occur. Cardiac failure didn't end my father's life even though this is what appears on his death certificate—an erroneously introduced MRSA bloodstream infection did.

---

*1998 Institute of Medicine, *To Err is Human: Building a Safer Health Care System*
2003 Healthgrades, *Patient Safety in American Hospitals*
2010 U.S. Department of Health and Human Services Office of Inspector General, *Adverse Events in Hospitals: National Incidence Among Medicare Beneficiaries*
** Patient Safety, Science & Technology Summit, 2015

Emergency Room dying
within the Abrupt timeframe
under Machine control

Control	Abrupt Dying	Medically managed Dying			Never-ending Dying
		Onset	Progressed	Endstage	
World	Sudden	Insleep			
Medical	Erroneous				
Machine	Emergency Room				
Personal					
Shared					

Most of us refer to the Emergency Department colloquially as the "ER," short for emergency room. Dying in an emergency room is Abrupt by definition. Although the use of life-support machinery is not an absolute, the likelihood is high that a life-and-death ER visit will include the use of life supports, thus this landing is under Machine control. Furthermore, first responders default to lifesaving measures. They will ignore extra-legal cues like do-not-recuscitate tattoos and are known to override legitimate proxy declarations against the medical rescue of a loved one. Stories circulate about elders a few days short of dying being transported to an emergency department (when all they needed was help getting back into bed) and ending up dying in-hospital several days later. Thus, this landing may be a way station en route to a harder landing of the type many people say they wish to avoid, as the emergency room's purpose is to stabilize people and move them out to other units in the hospital.

**Suicidal dying
within the Abrupt timeframe
under Personal control**

Control	Abrupt Dying	Medically managed Dying			Never-ending Dying
		Onset	Progressed	Endstage	
World	Sudden		Insleep		
Medical	Erroneous				
Machine	Emergency Room				
Personal	Suicidal				
Shared					

    The classic definition of suicide is to deliberately take one's own life, no matter the circumstances. Within Windrum's Matrix, Suicidal dying refers to non-terminal people ending their lives.

    People who favor the legalization of medical aid in dying (legalized physician assistance rendered when a person is dying of a terminal disease) distinguish between suicide, which takes a viable life, and self-deliverance when one is terminally ill and soon to die. People who oppose the legalization of aided dying suggest that any act of self-termination is suicide and that no further distinctions exist. We will address how the Matrix accounts for these differing viewpoints in the following chapter, Matrix: Ethics and Legalities.

Early dying
within the Medically managed Onset timeframe
under Medical control

Control	Abrupt Dying	Medically managed Dying			Never-ending Dying
		Onset	Progressed	Endstage	
World	Sudden	Insleep			
Medical	Erroneous	Early			
Machine	Emergency Room				
Personal	Suicidal				
Shared					

Early dying in the Onset timeframe under Medical control assumes fewer invasive medical treatments and less terminal decline to endure, hence a softer landing. Except for the very few people able to control their own trajectories and decide to die (without committing suicide), Early dying is not a landing we can aim for. It differs from the Abrupt timeframe because a terminal disease has emerged; it differs from World control because medicine has been engaged to treat the disease condition. Generally, we'd be surprised should someone experience Early dying.

Midstream dying
within the Medically managed Progressed timeframe under Medical control

Control	Abrupt Dying	Medically managed Dying			Never-ending Dying
		Onset	Progressed	Endstage	
World	Sudden		Insleep		
Medical	Erroneous	Early	Midstream		
Machine	Emergency Room				
Personal	Suicidal				
Shared					

Midstream dying simply means that one has moved through Early dying based on the passage of time and well-known markers of disease progression and does not live into a drawn-out endstage of disease.

Endstate dying
within the Medically managed Endstage timeframe
under Medical control

Control	Abrupt Dying	Medically managed Dying			Never-ending Dying
		Onset	Progressed	Endstage	
World	Sudden	Insleep			
Medical	Erroneous	Early	Midstream	Endstate	
Machine	Emergency Room				
Personal	Suicidal				
Shared					

Endstate dying means that one has sustained through to the very end of survivability; death will no longer occur as a surprise, rather it's expected, perhaps welcomed. Generally, expect Endstate dying to be a very hard landing.

SlowMotion dying
within the Never-ending timeframe
under World or Medical control

Control	Abrupt Dying	Medically managed Dying			Never-ending Dying
		Onset	Progressed	Endstage	
World	Sudden	Insleep			SlowMotion
Medical	Erroneous	Early	Midstream	Endstate	SlowMotion
Machine	Emergency Room				
Personal	Suicidal				
Shared					

SlowMotion dying under World or Medical controls refers to long, drawn-out demises. Any demise stretching into extreme timeframes—a new normal spanning long months or years—is Never-ending. Under World control, sufferers of cognitive decline and the various dementias manage to age with minimal or no medical intervention required. Dementia might be a sole illness or a comorbidity; it's a significant contributing factor to Never-ending dying. Under Medical control, the dying require ongoing medical treatments; engaging with the medical system will complicate their lives and the lives of their caregivers. With or without medical engagement, Never-ending dying typically taxes loved-ones-as-caregivers to extremes. In the worst cases, family wealth and caregiver health can be decimated, making the experience of SlowMotion dying severely demanding for all involved.

Delayed dying
within the Medically managed Onset timeframe
under Machine control

Control	Abrupt Dying	Medically managed Dying			Never-ending Dying
		Onset	Progressed	Endstage	
World	Sudden	Insleep			SlowMotion
Medical	Erroneous	Early	Midstream	Endstate	
Machine	Emergency Room	Delayed			
Personal	Suicidal				
Shared					

By definition, the moment life supports are introduced, dying has been delayed. Should death occur relatively soon after their introduction, within the onset of some terminal health condition being held at bay by those life supports, the patient-family experiences Delayed dying. Delayed dying shortly after the onset of disease could be viewed as cheatingly early, or it could be thought of as a blessing in disguise—limiting both the dying person's and their loved ones' exposure to longer and harder situations.

Suspended dying
within the Medically managed Progressed timeframe under Machine control

Control	Abrupt Dying	Medically managed Dying			Never-ending Dying
		Onset	Progressed	Endstage	
World	Sudden	Insleep			SlowMotion
Medical	Erroneous	Early	Midstream	Endstate	
Machine	Emergency Room	Delayed	Suspended		
Personal	Suicidal				
Shared					

Suspended dying under Machine control is one of several landings we have in mind when we fearfully envision hospitalized dying: connected to a range of life-support machinery where we've lain for some weeks. Benchmarks exist that inform medical professionals as to how long any individual may remain attached to different types of life supports; the more time passes, the more, and more invasive, the life supports that must be introduced. Suspended dying is a landing where, generally speaking, the less invasive life supports are applied (expect machine ventilation here but generally not a surgically inserted feeding tube). Suspended dying is an indeterminate place where the patient—and to some extent the family—are neither living nor dying.

I have experienced Suspended dying; my mother landed here after succumbing to sudden respiratory collapse, and we languished here for more than two weeks before removing her life support.

Repetitive dying
within the Medically managed Endstage timeframe
under Machine control

Control	Abrupt Dying	Medically managed Dying			Never-ending Dying
		Onset	Progressed	Endstage	
World	Sudden	Insleep			SlowMotion
Medical	Erroneous	Early	Midstream	Endstate	
Machine	Emergency Room	Delayed	Suspended	Repetitive	
Personal	Suicidal				
Shared					

The idea of dying moment to moment and being resuscitated moment by moment when attached to a breathing ventilator is poetic. Repetitive dying's extended duration of three to four weeks, be that wholly contained within this landing or the cumulative duration from neighboring landings, puts Repetitive dying in a league of its own. The futility quotient here informs this landing's almost mechanical name. It's a no person's land where normalcy absents itself and new existential rules apply. Repetitive is not technically accurate; the patient is not actually dying again and again. Loved ones languishing through long weeks may feel as if they are. The word "repetitive" is a wake-up call to those maintaining the unmaintainable upon a loved one who will not wake or walk this earth again.

Vegetative dying
within the Never-ending timeframe
under Machine control

Control	Abrupt Dying	Medically managed Dying			Never-ending Dying
		Onset	Progressed	Endstage	
World	Sudden		Insleep		SlowMotion
Medical	Erroneous	Early	Midstream	Endstate	
Machine	Emergency Room	Delayed	Suspended	Repetitive	Vegetative
Personal	Suicidal				
Shared					

Vegetative dying is the place where people who have traversed Suspended and Repetitive dying finally land, or where people who have survived Sudden dying may land when "saved" by first responders. The name refers to the condition known as "persistent vegetative state" or "permanent vegetative state." Technically, the vegetative condition is characterized by irreversible brain damage and unaware wakefulness; recently, a sensitivity toward referring to any person as a vegetable has stimulated a new descriptor, "unresponsive wakefulness syndrome."

Whereas people who land in SlowMotion dying may take years to end up in an ICU, most people experiencing Vegetative dying have graduated from ICUs to LTACs (long-term acute care facilities). LTAC facilities warehouse populations of bodies permanently attached to machines via surgically implanted breathing and feeding tubes. Vegetative dying refers to a body kept artificially alive for months to years; death is not allowed to occur. Since 1975, cases of this sort have made national news and stimulated laws when involved parties turn to the courts to sustain or remove life supports.

Released dying
within the Medically managed Onset timeframe
under Personal control

Control	Abrupt Dying	Medically managed Dying			Never-ending Dying
		Onset	Progressed	Endstage	
World	Sudden	Insleep			SlowMotion
Medical	Erroneous	Early	Midstream	Endstate	
Machine	Emergency Room	Delayed	Suspended	Repetitive	Vegetative
Personal	Suicidal	Released			
Shared					

Released dying refers to self-directed dying very soon after receiving a terminal diagnosis. If self-directed dying occurs within a nation or a U.S. state where medical aid in dying is legal and that process has been engaged, the dying will be state sanctioned. If self-directed dying occurs outside those jurisdictions or processes, the dying will be extra-legal. In order to experience Released dying, people must be very proactive, understanding laws, methods of self-deliverance, and manifesting readiness to act.

Postponed dying
within the Medically managed Progressed timeframe
under Personal control

Control	Abrupt Dying	Medically managed Dying			Never-ending Dying
		Onset	Progressed	Endstage	
World	Sudden		Insleep		SlowMotion
Medical	Erroneous	Early	Midstream	Endstate	
Machine	Emergency Room	Delayed	Suspended	Repetitive	Vegetative
Personal	Suicidal	Released	Postponed		
Shared					

Postponed dying is the landing for people who desire to live as long as possible before ending their lives under Personal control. Pathways include ingesting life-ending prescription medication through aided-dying laws, VSED (voluntarily stopping eating and drinking), or independent self-deliverance. Those utilizing aided dying will wait until they sense that if they wait longer they risk being unable to independently ingest the prescribed lethal medication as U.S. laws require.

Failed dying
within the Medically managed Endstage timeframe
under Personal control

Control	Abrupt Dying	Medically managed Dying			Never-ending Dying
		Onset	Progressed	Endstage	
World	Sudden	Insleep			SlowMotion
Medical	Erroneous	Early	Midstream	Endstate	
Machine	Emergency Room	Delayed	Suspended	Repetitive	Vegetative
Personal	Suicidal	Released	Postponed	Failed	
Shared					

People who land in Failed dying have waited too long and have lost the strength, coordination, or swallowing ability necessary to ingest lethal prescriptions. Perhaps they've waited too long to begin the application process and no longer meet the cognitive requirements or are unable to muster the stamina to find willing doctors and travel to meet with them for the required interviews. Failed dying is the most transitory, ephemeral landing because, by definition, those who land here cannot die here. They get immediately shifted into the hardest dying situations. For those who value aided dying or self-deliverance, landing in Failed dying is heartbreaking, the awful experience of promise pain.

Collaborative dying throughout the Medically managed timeframe under Shared control

Control	Abrupt Dying	Medically managed Dying			Never-ending Dying
		Onset	Progressed	Endstage	
World	Sudden	Insleep			SlowMotion
Medical	Erroneous	Early	Midstream	Endstate	
Machine	Emergency Room	Delayed	Suspended	Repetitive	Vegetative
Personal	Suicidal	Released	Postponed	Failed	
Shared	Collaborative				

Collaborative dying refers to proactively using palliative treatments and/or enrolling in hospice. These are distinctly different, partially related resources, widely misunderstood and narrowly funded. Collaborative dying does not mean waiting until the last few days of life to utilize palliative medicine or to enroll in hospice following extended detours through other landings. (That's how tours through our dying territory typically go, with most end-of-life traffic routing through Progressed and Endstage timeframes under Medical and Machine control.) Immersion in Collaborative dying, which offers a range of peace-inducing practical benefits for all involved, requires that landing here be more than an afterthought. Embracing Collaborative dying means engaging with it over an extended time, a minimum of some weeks and generally several months.

For societies in which social order is intact, as far as my thoughts are capable of going, these landings comprise the whole of our dying territory; there are no other dying situations. These landings function as way stations and final destinations within our dying territory. We, each and all, bring our varied circumstances to these landings—our outlooks, relationships, and resources; our strengths and weaknesses; our morbidities, fortunes, and destinies.

Chapter 7

Matrix: Ethics and Legalities

Windrum's Matrix of Dying Terms ™

Control	Abrupt Dying	Medically managed Dying			Never-ending Dying
		Onset	Progressed	Endstage	
World	Sudden	Insleep			SlowMotion
Medical	Erroneous	Early	Midstream	Endstate	
Machine	Emergency Room	Delayed	Suspended	Repetitive	Vegetative
Personal	Suicidal	Released	Postponed	Failed	
Shared		Collaborative			

LEGAL and/or ACCEPTED   ILLEGAL and/or UNACCEPTED   BOTH and/or AMBIGUOUS

This is the complete Matrix of Dying Terms.

Before we deepen our inquiry by examining vignettes that exemplify each landing, there's one more aspect that the Matrix addresses: how our societies view the experience of dying in each of these situations through both legal and moral lenses. The light gray color indicates that experiences within the majority of dying situations are legal and socially acceptable. The gray-blue blend indicates landings that may be illegal or viewed by some or many people as unacceptable. Note that this discussion applies specifically to the United States; readers in other countries may need to mentally adjust these aspects based on laws and mores where you live.

Legalities are generally clearcut; things are either legal or they aren't. By "accepted" and "unaccepted" I mean, by and large, by the mainstream.

The Matrix clearly shows that mainstream medical treatments are both legal and accepted across the dying spectrum. Even on the far end of time, Full Code ("do everything") is the default of both medicine and the law and also the expectation of many citizens. This is despite the potential for experiences and outcomes that may shock, horrify, offend, and do more harm than good. That our society (we, insurers, and our government) will pay for long-term advanced Medical and Machine treatments testifies to their acceptability. Contrast this with comparatively miserly or absent resources or insurance coverage for necessary, humane, at-home caregiving which, in many anecdotal cases, proves to be existentially and financially draining for family members who assume the caregiver role and pay all its costs, financial, physical, and emotional, out of their own resources.

Ethical issues arise when considering several dying situations, indicated by landings colored with gray-blue blends.

Suicidal Dying Under Personal Control

In the United States, suicide is no longer illegal in any state. For many people, both religious and nonreligious, suicide—taking one's own viable life—remains troubling at best and morally abhorrent at worst. (*Assisting* a suicide is illegal throughout the United States and can result in felony manslaughter or murder charges.) Yet there is a cohort that believes in complete individual freedom and that ending one's life anytime is a human right. This landing is blended gray-blue because what constitutes a morally abhorrent suicide differs between mutually exclusive traditional and contemporary viewpoints.

Those who value personal liberty at the end of life above other considerations feel that aided-dying laws serve too narrow a segment of the terminally ill; that the decision to end one's life when terminal should extend to people whose disease trajectories are terminal yet outside of the restrictions typically written into U.S. laws. Some people distinguish between non-terminal ("irrational") suicide—the self-taking of a viable life—and "rational suicide," the self-taking of a terminal life which happens to fall outside aided-dying's eligibility requirements (six-month terminal diagnosis, competency at the time of application, and ability to hold and ingest the drugs without assistance). Some people take exception to making these distinctions at all, considering them judgmental.

Released and Postponed Dying

At this writing, medical aid in dying is legal across much of North America: in six U.S. states plus Washington, D.C. (covering approximately one-sixth of all U.S. citizens) and throughout all of Canada. Under the statutes and court rulings, people ending their lives and the medical and pharmaceutical professionals involved are not engaging in nor assisting suicides and are exempt from prosecution. (To be clear with the use of language: aided dying is referred to by its opponents as "assisted suicide," a phrase that proponents of aided dying consider pejorative).

People living in jurisdictions with no aided-dying statutes who engage in self-directed dying under Personal control using "uncontrolled" illegal substances or inventive methods do so extra-legally; those assisting them risk prosecution.

Although aided dying is favored by roughly two-thirds of the population in the United States and has been decreed a universal right across Canada, some conservative lawmakers continue seeking ways to cripple aided dying despite its passage by undeniable-to-significant majorities or by judicial ruling. Opponents of aided dying seem steadfast in believing it to be fundamentally immoral. The Matrix acknowledges these divergent viewpoints by blending Released and Postponed dying gray-blue.

Given the advent of aided dying in North America, the notion of exerting Personal control over our dying may be gaining more broad-based acceptance, beyond statements made in the heat of a painful moment, perhaps tinged with bravado. Medicine seems to agree that people should influence their own demises and deaths. Control is bigger than influence. Control is where the influence rubber meets the end-of-life road, with individual dying people directing their own demises in ways that put their experience and desire ahead of medical or socio-political norms. Yet the reality is that control is shared to some degree: claimed by default by medicine, negotiated by patient-families and medicine, or demanded and protected by civilians.

When I developed Windrum's Matrix and delivered my TEDx-FoCo talk, I referenced what I heard as a particularly sour assertion by an Australian intensivist (critical care doctor), Peter Saul, in his 2011 TEDxNewy talk. He referred to aided dying, in Oregon and in general, as euthanasia and "a sideshow" that "doesn't matter" because aided-dying deaths account for a small percentage of all deaths. During my TEDx talk I responded, saying: "If the only... dying outcomes, of 17*, that potentially put dying under our Personal control are going to be called a 'sideshow,' then I think we need to ask, 'What is happening to millions of American families and more millions worldwide under the medical Big Top—and what is our role in that?'"

Aided dying matters greatly to those who desire to exercise Personal control, not just influence, over their dying. It matters to those who recognize the generations-long slope of overmedicalized

---

*At the time of the TEDx talk Windrum's Matrix contained 16 landings. I've written 17 here for consistency with this book's discussion.

dying and don't want to end their lives there. Assuming, that is, that they can qualify under these laws' narrow, restrictive terms.

Endstate and Repetitive Dying

All medical treatments applied in these landings are legal and accepted for those who choose to "do everything," no matter to what lengths or how protracted, no matter what harms may be delivered, no matter how torturous any outcome, with two exceptions...

First, gray-blue blending accounts for moral disquiet felt by those who find it abhorrent to sustain biological life to every length and any cost regardless of the futility of doing so or harm to the dying.

Second, what I call "wink-nod euthanasia," the painless killing of a suffering terminally-ill person; i.e., undocumented instances of an extra amount of morphine sent through the intravenous line to put a loved one out of his or her misery, and onlooking family members out of theirs. It's done intentionally by whichever medical professional adjusts the equipment, usually with the tacit approval of key family members on hand, communicated not in writing or with speech but by eye contact and subtle body language. Although well-known, I haven't seen data accounting for wink-nod euthanasia and don't expect to. The blended designation in the Endstate and Repetitive landings accounts for this quiet, often desired yet illegal euthanasia, which is widely viewed as ethical and moral, a blessed relief for the dying and their survivors. People just don't share this assessment openly.

Vegetative Dying

The warehousing of bodies kept alive by machinery, in some cases for years, is seen by some as a grotesque and offensive transfiguration of medicine. The practice is legal and available, and there can be no denying it as an unsettling seam in our social fabric. In American jurisprudence, vegetative cases have made historic law.

Chapter 8

Matrix: Landing Vignettes

Now that we've toured our dying territory, you may have questions about where on the Matrix your own previously experienced or imagined future scenarios might be situated. This chapter presents 17 vignettes that exemplify the nature of each dying situation. Each scenario is presented from the imagined perspective of a person who has died.

Earlier I made a distinction between situations and circumstances. I defined situations as being made up of circumstances. Matrix landings in which we find ourselves are our dying situations; circumstances do not define them. This is not to say that circumstances don't matter to us; they most certainly do. Many aspects of our lives influence how peacefully we die—which disease(s) we have; whether we are financially solvent or not; whether we have healthy or toxic family relationships; if religious beliefs are present or absent; how well or poorly we may be educated about medical matters. Our circumstances fill our landings when we enter; when we leave, our circumstances leave with us. Circumstances are not relevant to the job the Matrix does for us. The Matrix simply applies two cardinal aspects of dying—a timeline and a controlling entity—to identify common dying situations so that we may stand back, survey our dying territory, recognize its way stations, and ask, "Do I want to land there?" And then to ask, "What must I learn, what skills must I acquire, in order to increase my likelihood of attaining or avoiding these landings?" Asking and answering these questions can materially change the future circumstances you bring with you throughout your own or a loved one's demise.

The following 17 fictional (except as noted) vignettes depict circumstances and reflections associated with dying in each Matrix landing. In life there are a zillion variables; these vignettes present one example for each landing. In them the deceased speak to us from the beyond.

Control	Abrupt Dying	Medically managed Dying			Never-ending Dying
		Onset	Progressed	Endstage	
World	Sudden	Insleep			SlowMotion
Medical	Erroneous	Early	Midstream	Endstate	
Machine	Emergency Room	Delayed	Suspended	Repetitive	Vegetative
Personal	Suicidal	Released	Postponed	Failed	
Shared		Collaborative			

Insleep dying

Having reached 74 years of age, I was "winding down" a bit but felt relatively healthy. One night I went to sleep and never woke up again. I, like many, had vocalized how Insleep dying would be my preferred way to go, but I never expected I'd win this end-of-life lottery. Although most people don't, I experienced Insleep dying. My loved ones experienced my Insleep dying, too. I'm sorry my remains shocked my wife when she awoke next to me. Seeing my body in bed was shocking for my other family members too. With time they came to consider my death to have been as gentle for them as it was for me, especially compared to the experiences of so many others with drawn-out deaths in harder landings.

Control	Abrupt Dying	Medically managed Dying			Never-ending Dying
		Onset	Progressed	Endstage	
World	Sudden	Insleep			SlowMotion
Medical	Erroneous	Early	Midstream	Endstate	
Machine	Emergency Room	Delayed	Suspended	Repetitive	Vegetative
Personal	Suicidal	Released	Postponed	Failed	
Shared		Collaborative			

Sudden dying

I'm not alive anymore! I experienced Sudden dying. It happened instantly. It was a lightning strike—literally a bolt out of the blue (although when we imagined Sudden dying, we spoke of events that felt more likely to occur, like a car wreck or an earthquake or a gunshot or an instantly fatal heart attack). My surviving loved ones who were next to me witnessed, and in so doing experienced, my Sudden dying, too. The trauma they experienced was entirely of the World's making.

Control	Abrupt Dying	Medically managed Dying			Never-ending Dying
		Onset	Progressed	Endstage	
World	Sudden	Insleep			SlowMotion
Medical	Erroneous	Early	Midstream	Endstate	
Machine	Emergency Room	Delayed	Suspended	Repetitive	Vegetative
Personal	Suicidal	Released	Postponed	Failed	
Shared		Collaborative			

Erroneous dying

I underwent pacemaker eligibility testing as a hospital outpatient. My family and I made an error in judgement—the chemical test overstressed my heart; I crashed medically and was admitted to the hospital. I acquired a preventable, hospital-caused urinary tract MRSA superbug infection through a urinary catheter. The infection migrated to my bloodstream and painfully lodged in a wrist, causing debilitation and widespread sepsis that I could not overcome. My hospitalized demise took about two weeks. The death certificate says, "congestive heart failure," but I know better—it should read "medical error." I and my loved ones experienced Erroneous dying. It was a hard landing for all of us. (The true story of my father's demise)

Control	Abrupt Dying	Medically managed Dying			Never-ending Dying
		Onset	Progressed	Endstage	
World	Sudden	Insleep			SlowMotion
Medical	Erroneous	Early	Midstream	Endstate	
Machine	Emergency Room	Delayed	Suspended	Repetitive	Vegetative
Personal	Suicidal	Released	Postponed	Failed	
Shared		Collaborative			

Emergency Room dying

We were so old. My wife was 87, I was 91 and dying. We did everything we had been advised, all the directives including the POLST directive declining all life-support measures. At 3 o'clock in the morning I fell on my way back to bed from the bathroom, and we couldn't get me off the floor. My wife panicked and called 911. All she wanted was for them to lift me back into bed, but, despite our directives and pleas, they whisked me off to the Emergency Room—the last place on Earth I'd wanted to go. I was so frail that the mayhem precipitated another heart episode. Since we didn't have my directives with us they called Full Code on me, a full-court press to try to prevent my dying. My wife was so distraught. I died under assault, exactly the opposite of what we thought we'd carefully planned. If I hadn't died in the ER, the overwhelming likelihood is that I would've died in an ICU several days later—the whole episode making it physically impossible for me to return home. Thing is, we never asked ourselves if it was OK to die on the floor between the bed and the wall. Would it have been? My loved ones in the waiting room witnessed the mayhem being done to my diminished body. I wish they hadn't. I wish I hadn't, too. All our planning... for naught. (Based on a true story)

Control	Abrupt Dying	Medically managed Dying			Never-ending Dying
		Onset	Progressed	Endstage	
World	Sudden	Insleep			SlowMotion
Medical	Erroneous	Early	Midstream	Endstate	
Machine	Emergency Room	Delayed	Suspended	Repetitive	Vegetative
Personal	Suicidal	Released	Postponed	Failed	
Shared		Collaborative			

Suicidal dying

I had no physical disease. I was not elderly. I was not terminally ill. I had my problems, which loomed larger to me than yours do to you. So I took to the bridge. I'm a statistic now. Aw, all my details don't matter. I ended my life by my own hand. My loved ones may or may not understand my reasons.

Control	Abrupt Dying	Medically managed Dying			Never-ending Dying
		Onset	Progressed	Endstage	
World	Sudden	Insleep			SlowMotion
Medical	Erroneous	Early	Midstream	Endstate	
Machine	Emergency Room	Delayed	Suspended	Repetitive	Vegetative
Personal	Suicidal	Released	Postponed	Failed	
Shared		Collaborative			

Early dying

Almost nobody plans to die so very soon after receiving a formal terminal diagnosis (when the docs don't think you'll be alive at the end of six months' time). But I did; I dropped off two weeks later. Am I lucky? I'd been feeling totally worn out; my organs and systems didn't respond to any therapy. They called it "failure to thrive." During my second day in our elder community's nursing facility, my body just had enough. That I died so soon after being pronounced terminal was traumatic for my loved ones. But the flip side is that due to the short duration of my demise, little if any additional traumas—the kind arising from protracted, ultimately futile medical treatments—added to their loss. They came to feel that we all lucked out by landing within Early dying.

Control	Abrupt Dying	Medically managed Dying			Never-ending Dying
		Onset	Progressed	Endstage	
World	Sudden	Insleep			SlowMotion
Medical	Erroneous	Early	**Midstream**	Endstate	
Machine	Emergency Room	Delayed	Suspended	Repetitive	Vegetative
Personal	Suicidal	Released	Postponed	Failed	
Shared		Collaborative			

Midstream dying

In the hospital again…. I'd lost track of how many times during the six months since we first knew that there were no cures for my ailments. During the last several months, my conditions had improved and declined and improved again, like a roller coaster. But one day I finally turned for the worse. I arrived the last time with several comorbidities. We stuck it out in-hospital, trying this and that intervention rather than bailing on my loved ones' hopes for my cure and restoration. One early morning seven days into this hospitalization, I died. I didn't get out of Dodge particularly quickly, but my loved ones feel fortunate that I, and they, were spared the most invasive, hard-to-bear medical interventions. I died Midstream, neither surprisingly soon, nor agonizingly protracted.

Control	Abrupt Dying	Medically managed Dying			Never-ending Dying
		Onset	Progressed	Endstage	
World	Sudden	Insleep			SlowMotion
Medical	Erroneous	Early	Midstream	Endstate	
Machine	Emergency Room	Delayed	Suspended	Repetitive	Vegetative
Personal	Suicidal	Released	Postponed	Failed	
Shared		Collaborative			

Endstate dying

I never knew which of my late-life hospitalizations would be my last. I never dreamt that the last one would last so long. More than a month, up and down, with every intervention at medicine's disposal. Should an 87-year-old subject herself to this? Had those treatments stretched any further, I would've become a vegetable. Mine was a hard death for everyone because none of us considered allowing an easier one. I still don't know why we were so reluctant to allow death to come; truth be told I was ready, and it had been knocking at my door for the last year of my life. So we ran out the clock, insisting that "everything be done." Back and forth to hospitals and rehab joints; the last ambulance ride was straight to the ICU. I went Full Code and they all jumped my bones even as my body was trying its best to die. So we all experienced Endstate dying, and all I know is that some of my kids wished we hadn't, because that's what they will remember, always.

Control	Abrupt Dying	Medically managed Dying			Never-ending Dying
		Onset	Progressed	Endstage	
World	Sudden	Insleep			SlowMotion
Medical	Erroneous	Early	Midstream	Endstate	
Machine	Emergency Room	Delayed	Suspended	Repetitive	Vegetative
Personal	Suicidal	Released	Postponed	Failed	
Shared		Collaborative			

SlowMotion dying

I've succumbed to cognitive decline. It's been more than six years, during which I've had several strokes, each one leaving me more debilitated. Now I can't do things even a child can. I can't bathe or dress, and I often forget how to eat. My spouse and adult children are sapped and drained, showing symptoms of traumatic stress. My wife hasn't had a day or week off in years. In my few lucid moments I wonder if she's not worse off than I am. I had hoped to bestow my children with my life savings but the money's all been spent because I need full-time assistance from the moment I wake up to the moment I fall asleep. I haven't died yet. This is SlowMotion dying. It seems to never end.

Control	Abrupt Dying	Medically managed Dying			Never-ending Dying
		Onset	Progressed	Endstage	
World	Sudden	Insleep			SlowMotion
Medical	Erroneous	Early	Midstream	Endstate	
Machine	Emergency Room	Delayed	Suspended	Repetitive	Vegetative
Personal	Suicidal	Released	Postponed	Failed	
Shared		Collaborative			

Delayed dying

The medical conditions I'd managed for years finally became comorbidities. Ever frailer, I don't even remember what landed me in the hospital—where they started trying to fix the unfixable. Within several days a jugular catheter was placed and dialysis started—my advance directive denying these treatments had not been entered into my chart, apparently lost between the admission desk and the nurses' station on my floor. The moment dialysis began my dying was delayed, life force replaced by machine. My spouse and children, my healthcare agents, produced my directive and demanded that the dialysis catheter be removed. I died a day later. Some doctors were aghast, but my family did right by me.

Control	Abrupt Dying	Medically managed Dying			Never-ending Dying
		Onset	Progressed	Endstage	
World	Sudden	Insleep			SlowMotion
Medical	Erroneous	Early	Midstream	Endstate	
Machine	Emergency Room	Delayed	Suspended	Repetitive	Vegetative
Personal	Suicidal	Released	Postponed	Failed	
Shared		Collaborative			

Suspended dying

I was in the waiting room of an outpatient clinic when I suddenly couldn't breathe and accepted help. Apparently, I crashed completely because that help became a breathing tube. The docs called it treatment, but it morphed into life support; I never regained consciousness. Despite advance directives that intended otherwise, my family pursued a treatment course lasting weeks. At the end, it took several days to get the ventilator removed. I died several hours later in the ICU. The staff was so callous that no one came to turn off the alarms. My daughter sat alone with my body; eventually she figured out how to turn the alarms off herself. My family and I experienced the Neverland of Suspended dying for almost three interminable weeks. They wish we hadn't. They'll never un-experience it. (The true story of my mother's demise)

Control	Abrupt Dying	Medically managed Dying			Never-ending Dying
		Onset	Progressed	Endstage	
World	Sudden	Insleep			SlowMotion
Medical	Erroneous	Early	Midstream	Endstate	
Machine	Emergency Room	Delayed	Suspended	**Repetitive**	Vegetative
Personal	Suicidal	Released	Postponed	Failed	
Shared	Collaborative				

Repetitive dying

I've been intubated for a week beyond what safe medical practice supports. Unwilling to let me go, my family authorized a tracheostomy—a breathing tube surgically implanted through my neck, and also a PEG feeding tube sewn through my abdomen. This stuff doesn't come out as long as the body still "lives." There's no way outta here; this is the very end of the slippery slope that I'd said I never wanted to be on in the first place. My family cannot bring themselves to remove the tubes; it's so easy to put them in and so hard to pull them out. Here I remain, so far gone that I'm essentially dying every moment yet being resuscitated puff by puff, drip by drip, again and again. No one's said "vegetative" yet, but this must be close. Rinse and repeat, rinse and repeat, rinse and repeat…. Who's paying for this, anyway?

Control	Abrupt Dying	Medically managed Dying			Never-ending Dying
		Onset	Progressed	Endstage	
World	Sudden	Insleep			SlowMotion
Medical	Erroneous	Early	Midstream	Endstate	
Machine	Emergency Room	Delayed	Suspended	Repetitive	Vegetative
Personal	Suicidal	Released	Postponed	Failed	
Shared	Collaborative				

Vegetative dying

My dementia started 10 years ago when I was 76. My high blood pressure spiked precipitously post-op after a hip replacement at age 79. That landed us Midstream in Medically managed dying, fortunately as a way station. Over the next seven years the usual combination of ailments wore me down; I was in and out of hospitals and rehab as both an outpatient and inpatient. At age 86, acute pain associated with kidney failure landed me there this last time. After the stress of hospital-induced elder delirium, a stroke cut off the oxygen to my brain; now they say I'm brain dead. My body would shut down if only they'd let it. Somebody wanted everything done, and I failed to execute advance directives forbidding all the medical intervention I'm receiving. I even outlived my welcome in the ICU—I've been moved to a "long-term acute care facility." I've got both a breathing and feeding tube surgically sewn into me, and here I lie, warehoused with dozens of others like me. It's been four months since anyone other than doctors or nurses has come by to see me; my spouse is too frail to be driven even moderate distances and my adult children live far away. My body will never die unless they opt to not treat this new pneumonia or the power goes out. This building is filled with the remains of people on interminable life support. Maybe the power will go out, maybe it won't. If I could wonder, I would wonder what these years, past and future, are like for my loved ones. Did we intend to land here?

Control	Abrupt Dying	Medically managed Dying			Never-ending Dying
		Onset	Progressed	Endstage	
World	Sudden	Insleep			SlowMotion
Medical	Erroneous	Early	Midstream	Endstate	
Machine	Emergency Room	Delayed	Suspended	Repetitive	Vegetative
Personal	Suicidal	Released	Postponed	Failed	
Shared		Collaborative			

Released dying

I was 87. My disease got terminal and I was given a four-to-six months prognosis. My spouse had predeceased me several years ago. I was intent upon not doing anything that would introduce the risk of being placed on life-support machines. My life had been full: my failures legion, my accomplishments many. I had no need to linger. I had long since filled out, signed, and had witnessed my aided-dying application form. My doctor had assured me she would work with me through this legal process. She kept her word, and I bought the prescribed lethal medication. I held a final soirée with my few remaining friends and family, then mixed and ingested the "cocktail." My caregivers still had a few last-minute details to manage, but I died peacefully several hours later, where and how I chose. All of us, myself and my loved ones, were Released.

Control	Abrupt Dying	Medically managed Dying			Never-ending Dying
		Onset	Progressed	Endstage	
World	Sudden	Insleep			SlowMotion
Medical	Erroneous	Early	Midstream	Endstate	
Machine	Emergency Room	Delayed	Suspended	Repetitive	Vegetative
Personal	Suicidal	Released	**Postponed**	Failed	
Shared		Collaborative			

Postponed dying

I was 72 with stage 4 terminal cancer. It was rough, but we managed the pain with good palliative care, medical marijuana, and hospice. My large family was a joy, and several of my adult children returned to share my remaining time at our home. I had no desire or need to go sooner. These last three months were difficult, yet a blessing; I'd seen and bid farewell to everyone. Time passed; I postponed my dying. I took the life-ending prescription at the moment right for me, dying completely in, and at, peace. I lived as fully as I was able to throughout my demise. My loved ones, though sad, have happy memories of my final months on Earth.

Control	Abrupt Dying	Medically managed Dying			Never-ending Dying
		Onset	Progressed	Endstage	
World	Sudden	Insleep			SlowMotion
Medical	Erroneous	Early	Midstream	Endstate	
Machine	Emergency Room	Delayed	Suspended	Repetitive	Vegetative
Personal	Suicidal	Released	Postponed	Failed	
Shared		Collaborative			

Failed dying

I had ALS—Lou Gehrig's progressively debilitating disease. As a rural veterinarian, I'd euthanized many large animals. I had vowed to deliver myself before losing the ability to do so, but I let my family prevail upon me not to. I ended up immobile, capable of absolutely nothing—nothing at all. I could not change position, dress or undress, hold a glass, raise it to my mouth, or even swallow a cupful of anything. So I failed to qualify for aided dying under the terms of any U.S. aided-dying law. I can't believe it. Postponed dying was within my reach; Failed dying booted me across the dying territory to Repetitive dying. My death was hard and drawn-out to a most bitter end—an end I had promised to save myself from. And I failed. (Based on a true story)

Control	Abrupt Dying	Medically managed Dying			Never-ending Dying
		Onset	Progressed	Endstage	
World	Sudden	Insleep			SlowMotion
Medical	Erroneous	Early	Midstream	Endstate	
Machine	Emergency Room	Delayed	Suspended	Repetitive	Vegetative
Personal	Suicidal	Released	Postponed	Failed	
Shared		Collaborative			

Collaborative dying

I arranged early for palliative treatment and subsequently enrolled with a well-chosen hospice as soon as the docs declared me terminal. Not all hospices are created equal; we found a good one. Once we ironed out staffing issues, with hospice's help I was able to stay at home, although the hospice we selected had a small residential facility for people needing more intensive oversight than adult children or aged friends could provide. My demise had been reasonably well managed, and I used the time to orient spiritually. My loved ones and I had crucial medical and daily-living support when we needed it, and hospice helped them process my demise and passing—that's part of their job. I died peacefully, although not in full control. I'm happy that we found professional medical help oriented toward dying in peace when incurably terminal; we avoided the pressure to subject ourselves to late-life medical heroics. If I were still in the world, I would crow about Collaborative dying from the treetops, but I'm at peace among the tree roots now.

Chapter 9

Matrix: Guided Recitation
Trying Each Landing On For Size

"I Might Experience..."

Thus far I've presented, and you've received, information mind-to-mind. Unless, that is, something that's passed between us has triggered an emotional response, causing a catch in your heart, a lump in your throat, or a tear in your eye—all of which I've experienced repeatedly in the course of developing this work. I trust that you find the value I do in conceiving of the range of dying situations ahead of us as a territory with way stations and final landings that we can aim for or aim away from, assuming enough time and knowledge to do so (acquiring that knowledge is the subject of this book's last chapters).

Windrum's Matrix offers us a gateway to peaceful dying, and at this juncture we are imaginatively standing just inside it. In this chapter we'll venture deeper into our dying territory. Here we will get out of our heads and into our hearts, guts, and souls.

During live presentations of Windrum's Matrix, I lead groups through a guided recitation. We speak aloud together, "I might experience xyz dying." We recite this 17 times, substituting for "xyz" each landing name in turn. After the group recites each landing name, I take a few moments to extemporaneously pose questions and offer reflections on the possibility of our lives ending within that landing.

MATRIX GUIDED RECITATION

Insofar as printed pages allow, let's do that now. If you're alone, you'll speak each statement aloud, then read my reflections about them. *Allow your pace to slow.*

These reflections were transcribed from my spoken stream of thought, intoned at a contemplative pace. They are one-offs; each recitation is a unique improvisation. The recitations include factual, lyrical, and poetic elements inquiring into existential aspects of each projected experience.

If you're with others, speak each statement aloud together, then read each reflection aloud. You might consider a second pass through the "I might experience…" statements, substituting your stream-of-consciousness reflections for mine. What statements you make and questions you pose might prove illuminating! If you're reciting with a group, you might take turns offering reflections on the landings. As an alternative to reading the recitation, an audio file is available at AxiomAction.com/recitation-audio where you may recite along with me in a one-on-one session. To access the password-protected page, enter "RecitationAudio#".

Engaging with this chapter this way should take between 20 and 30 minutes for a single pass through the recitation, or as long as your own musings may require.

As you proceed, notice how you respond to the possibility of experiencing each dying situation, each Matrix landing. Perhaps some landing names will resonate with particular force, positively or negatively. Notice cues from your body. If speaking aloud the name of a particular dying situation induces cringes—or feels so distasteful that you don't even want to say it—that's a reliable indicator that you might want to learn a lot about how to decrease your likelihood of experiencing that dying situation. If speaking aloud the name of another landing relaxes you, you might want to learn how to increase your likelihood of reaching that place.

And, if due to a loved one's prior death, the mention of some landing makes you want to pause, go ahead and do so. Those of us with painful memories know how durable they are, how little it takes to reanimate them. Should the need to pause arise, honor it; feelings are allowed and encouraged. If you're with a group, after completing this tour of our dying territory, allow time to discuss aspects of the experience that may arise.

During presentations, I display each landing name on a screen and speak the name. I raise one or both index fingers as if I were conducting an orchestra and on the imaginary downbeat we recite together. First, we do a dry run, hearing ourselves and setting a pace. Here's your dry run; use it as a lead-in to the recitation. First say the name, then recite the "I might…" statement. Take your time.

PEACEFUL

[recite]   "I might experience Peaceful dying."

PEACE-LESS

[recite]   "I might experience Peace-less dying."

PEACEFUL

[recite]   "I might experience Peaceful dying."

Now, let's tour our dying territory, trying each landing on for size.

INSLEEP

[recite]   "I might experience Insleep dying"

[reflect] ...*throughout the Medically managed timeframe under World control. Widely held to be the Holy Grail of dying experiences. Many say, "I want to die in my sleep." If you do is that okay? Are you okay with dying unconsciously? Or, do you want to consciously experience your death? If you were to die in your sleep would you come to on the other side, at the entrance to the Underworld, feeling cheated, and say so to Orpheus?*

Insleep dying.

SUDDEN

[recite]   "I might experience Sudden dying"

[reflect]   ...*in the Abrupt timeframe under World control. What would do me in? A heart attack? A car crash? A tornado? A bullet? We have no say with Sudden dying—Sudden dying speaks conclusively.*

Sudden dying.

ERRONEOUS

[recite]   "I might experience Erroneous dying."

[reflect]   ...in the Abrupt timeframe under Medical control. Abrupt because the moment of error—be it poor judgment or medical mistake—changes one's trajectory irrevocably. The Erroneous landing is strange; we land for a moment in a way station that projects us across our dying territory to some other landing where we do not want to be. What leads to circumstances in which misadventure or error might arise? Did we place ourselves in those circumstances? Did we roll the dice one too many times? Did we make a prudent choice? Was the promise of medical treatment worth risking our peaceful demise?

Erroneous dying.

EMERGENCY ROOM

[recite]   "I might experience Emergency Room dying."

[reflect]   *...in the Abrupt timeframe under Machine control. And how did I get here? Who made the call? Was my trip here of worldly origin? Was my trip here because a stranger made the call? Was my trip here a result of my repeat quest for More Time?*

Emergency Room dying.

SUICIDAL

[recite] "I might experience Suicidal dying."

[reflect] ...in the Abrupt timeframe under Personal control. And why would I have done that? Was my suicide rational—the taking of a long lived and completed life? Was my suicide of pain and angst; the shortening of a life already too short; the loss of a self so dear to others unable to help?

Suicidal dying.

EARLY

[recite] "I might experience Early dying."

[reflect] ...in the Medically managed Onset timeframe under Medical control. And if I do, ought I count my blessings? Granted, it might be unusual to die early after a formal terminal diagnosis due to the onset of a morbid disease. Have we control? Could we will ourselves to death as a strategy, as a pathway to navigate the mainstream of our dying territory, traveling down and stepping off the boat, onto the banks of the River Styx before reaching its rapids?

Early dying.

MIDSTREAM

[recite]   "I might experience Midstream dying."

[reflect]   ...*in the Medically managed Progressed timeframe under Medical control... which might make me somewhat ordinary. A disease, or several conditions having progressed through a reasonable time. Conventional medical treatments; abatement; attempts to forestall; it's tolerable, not having gone too far...*

Midstream dying.

ENDSTATE

[recite]   "I might experience Endstate dying."

[reflect]   *...in the Medically managed Endstage timeframe under Medical control. I the dying and my loved ones would traverse the full breadth of this landing, the endstate of the endstage. Those who value battle may join it here. This will be a hard landing. So hard that some might request, and be silently offered, the push of the plunger, an ambiguous assist under the auspices of an ethical construct called the Principle of Double Effect. This is one of several landings that many or most of us say that we do not want to visit! And so, what exactly would facilitate our not visiting? How could we aim away from Endstate dying? What must we know? What must we foresee? What must we forecast to minimize our likelihood of landing here?*

Endstate dying.

SLOWMOTION

[recite]   "I might experience SlowMotion dying."

[reflect]   ...*in the Never-ending timeframe under World or Medical control. Would the world do this to me? Of course it would! In this age of commonplace medical miracles that grant us all so much precious life, we're outliving our own brains. What an amazement! And truly, would medicine do this to me? Of course it would, if we let it—because SlowMotion dying is an extreme landing. Unlike under World control, here under Medical control we are aged bodies with failing minds. If the World isn't done with us, medicine won't be either. Remnants; a poignant conundrum for all.*

SlowMotion dying.

DELAYED

[recite]   "I might experience Delayed dying."

[reflect]   *...in the Medically managed Onset timeframe under Machine control. The moment life support begins, one's dying has been delayed. In many ways and some instances life supports are medical treatments, short-term miracles; we leave and we go home. When we are aged, when we are terminal and we have been placed on life support, we have entered the Matrix's Delayed landing—the place where we might really want to know our business. Is this the slippery slope? Is this where we lose our footing? Where we meet our maker before tumbling further?*

Delayed dying.

SUSPENDED

[recite]   "I might experience Suspended dying."

[reflect] ...*in the Medically managed Progressed timeframe under Machine control. This place of indetermination occupies a disproportionately large space across our dying territory. We who have landed here do not need statistics; its machines create statistics by recording us. Here in the middle of Windrum's Matrix is the sadly beating heart of our end-of-life troubles. This landing stretches on; our time here drags on; our emotions here press on our hearts; here our spirits need repair. Neither living nor dying, unable to set foot outside this landing, we stay too long, unable to set foot outside this landing...*

Suspended dying.

REPETITIVE

[recite]   "I might experience Repetitive dying."

[reflect]   ...*in the Medically managed Endstage timeframe under Machine control. At some point if we do not volunteer to set foot beyond Suspended dying we will involuntarily enter Repetitive dying. It's a subtle distinction, but I'll make it. An existential place of reimagination where in effect we die each moment, resuscitated by life supports each moment, again and again and again. And here, too, occasionally conflicted and kind-hearted people may silently lock eyes and say "Enough is enough, just a touch more through the IV, please." For those who do not lock eyes, say that Repetitive dying is the hardest of the hard...*

Repetitive dying.

VEGETATIVE

[recite]   "I might experience Vegetative dying."

[reflect]   *...in the Never-ending timeframe under Machine control... which in many, if not most, circumstances means that a body is warehoused in some place dedicated to warehousing bodies, all of whom are not expected back amongst us. Sewn-in life supports. Maybe, at best, perpetual 24/7/365 team-based home care. Can we make sense of such a place?*

Vegetative dying.

RELEASED

[recite]   "I might experience Released dying."

[reflect]   *...in the Medically managed Onset timeframe under Personal control. Wow. WOW! There are places where the citizenry has enacted laws, however flawed, granting the potential for Released dying. It's a narrow space to slip through, a rent in the fabric of living and dying. For those to whom it's available, it's a blessed release. Where legal it's called aided dying and where not, well, people will be inventive. Is this for you? Perhaps, if you're terminally ill and have completed living. Here we may exercise personal volition in a profound and absolute way at and over the end of our lives.*

Released dying.

POSTPONED

[recite]   "I might experience Postponed dying."

[reflect] ...in the Medically managed Progressed timeframe under Personal control. And if I do, under the same legal circumstances as Released dying, or under extra-legal circumstances, then I have gone the distance, having lived life putting up with the diseases that have done me in, consciously using my More Time, waiting until I could literally not wait anymore; grateful for the assistance of modern medicine or my own moxie, bidding "fare ye well" to a life well-lived and to people well-loved.

Postponed dying.

FAILED

[recite] "I might experience Failed dying."

[reflect] ...*in the Medically managed Endstage timeframe under Personal control... which is both the truth and a lie. This is a queer landing, for if we value and purport to exercise Personal control over our dying, and we wait too long and cannot do it and so fail, oh this is the ultimate promise pain. For here we cannot act and we cannot act; we cannot act, we have failed. And it's a queer landing because we do not die here; Failed dying kicks us immediately into Endstate or Repetitive dying, and we have chosen this. Some do, who succumb to pleas from loved ones. Beware.*

Failed dying.

COLLABORATIVE

[recite]   "I might experience Collaborative dying."

[reflect]   *...in any timeframe within Medically managed dying under Shared control. What a concept! Here's hope for a better way of death. Still fraught with risk of misadventure, yet with promise for the best in all of us, brought to our most sacred time. With the potential to satisfy the sensibilities of the many participating sectors in our strangely constructed society. With the potential for as much comfort as is comfortably possible; the potential for peace, as we know how to find and maintain peace. Hopefully, you'll find it here...*

Collaborative dying.

PEACE-LESS

[recite]   "I might experience Peace-less dying."

[reflect]   ...and if I do, what range of circumstances could afflict me so? Could I not foresee disagreement among my family members? That conflicting beliefs would disrupt my surrogate's abilities? Did our inadequate finances play a part? We certainly had no words to adequately describe the death I died, the protracted stressful situation—or any language, for that matter, to functionally describe a death I might find acceptable. Why didn't we think to assess and give weight to all my prior life-threatening hospitalizations—did I really need to be the hero yet again? Heck, I thought that that old Living Will should have prevented more heroics; why didn't it? Why didn't it protect me from risky treatments that became snafus, forcing me into yet another hospitalization? A hospitalization, like the others, that my loved ones just weren't up to learning how to manage—so they didn't learn and didn't manage. And so, the treatments wore on while I wore out. And all the while there was no easily accessible way to learn any of this in enough time, before this last hurrah...

Peace-less dying.

PEACEFUL

[recite] "I might experience Peaceful dying."

[reflect] *...and if I do, what did I do to have increased my likelihood of dying in peace, and of dying at peace? Allow me to tell all my surviving loved ones from here, the beyond, the coordinates for peaceful dying, that they might so engage in a manner suitable for their circumstances. We wish every sentient being as pleasing a journey as is possible across their dying territory.*

Peaceful dying.

This concludes *The Promised Landing*'s core presentation, a proposed solution to the trouble we experience in the absence of identifying and naming everyday dying situations. The trouble is that without names, we can't account for situations that await us. We don't consider them, plan for them, or act in advance to mitigate their worst effects. As too many of us have learned, too many end-of-life situations cause deleterious effects on people who want to die in peace and on their surviving loved ones who want to remember them as having done so.

This obstacle to peaceful dying is part of a greater whole, the first of seven obstacles in my end-of-life worldview, any one of which can put the kibosh on our desire to die in peace, and every one of which we can mitigate and even overcome.

If your curiosity is piqued and you'd like to learn about the other prevalent obstacles to peaceful dying and consider some solutions, the rest of *The Promised Landing* lies ahead. I hope that you, like me, will find an upside in deeply investigating a topic with many downsides. I have found that the process of untangling and debugging what obstructed my family's path toward peaceful dying, not once but twice, has been empowering. It's given me hope that offsets my trepidation about future demises in my family.

While the lexicon accounts for all impediments, it cannot address all their particulars, for trouble can appear in many guises. At the risk of being trite, I will say that by deconstructing the worldly obstacles to peaceful dying, we begin making lemonade of lemons. We can moderate dying's bitterness by understanding our system, strengthening our ability to act in advance when possible and in the moment when necessary.

Obstacles to Peaceful Dying and How to Mitigate Them

To Die in Peace: Our Rights of Passage

Chapter 10

To Die In Peace—Our Rights of Passage

My parents' hospitalized deaths unsettled me deeply. For my own well-being, I had to untangle and "debug" the many harmful aspects we didn't foresee or understand and to which we succumbed. Those insights, detailed in my first book, *Notes from the Waiting Room: Managing a Loved One's End-of-Life Hospitalization*, are included and extended in a view of modern dying that I call To Die in Peace: Our Rights of Passage. This program addresses a range of problems that arise through engagement with the medical system, especially involving hospitalization, and even more so in an end-of-life context. (Other authors, both civilian and professional, examine additional important topics such as understanding the process of decline through new conceptual frameworks; finding and navigating late-life services; personally recording and charting a loved one's hospital stay and treatments; how doctors are coming to recognize and attempting to change toxic aspects of medical culture; and availing oneself of self-deliverance options.)

In To Die in Peace: Our Rights of Passage, I use "rights," not "rites." Rites are defined as "religious or solemn ceremonies." Last Rites are administered to subjects who lie passive and depleted. While end-of-life rites support spiritual calm, in no way are rites tools to manage obstacles to peaceful dying that await us throughout our dying territory.

Rights are a prerogative to which we are entitled—a birthright. We act upon rights to manifest them in our lives. Rights legitimize our choices. End-of-life rights legitimize us as advanced sentient beings, to whom our own deaths rightly belong. We could refer to the unencumbered possibility of achieving a peaceful demise as our deathright.

Human beings may claim a deathright—the right to die in peace and at peace. I don't mean that these rights are conferred by the universe; the universe owes us nothing. But the societies we've constructed owe us a reasonable opportunity to find peace throughout our dying time, without undue infringement, simply as a condition of being alive. Medical and social conventions as they have developed since the late-20th century (which in the USA are in large part a result of predatory Capitalism) make finding and experiencing end-of-life peace too hard for too many of us. For-profit medicine; a medical culture that defaults to a never-say-die approach to the end of life; federal reimbursement schemes that routinely pay for expensive surgical procedures and rarely if ever pay for inexpensive everyday needs (negatively impacting the dying and their caretakers, almost always at-home family members); and our own aversion to dying and death conspire to foist harder dying than is necessary on too many of us, over too many generations' time.

Yet rights must be claimed. Rights are not free, especially rights pertaining to life's most profound moments in societies inclined to treat us brusquely when common sense and decency suggest compassion and delicacy. Responsibilities are the corollary of rights. Unless we are lucky—right place, right time, right vibe, right karma—it's likely that each of us will have to do some sustained work in order to increase our likelihood of dying in peace.

This chapter describes the obstacles about which I offer guidance. Some of the discussion below may clarify what you need to know to sufficiently prepare for a given obstacle. However, mitigating or overcoming several of the obstacles will require significant time, effort, and reading beyond this book. In particular, learning how to advocate effectively during any medical encounter, especially challenging ones, is a broad personal endeavor.

I have identified 10 obstacles to dying in peace. Three—family relations, beliefs, and finances—are completely personal. When they arise, they can be deeply divisive and disruptive. I do not address how to manage them, but they're prevalent and influential and so must be mentioned. About the other seven obstacles I offer a lot, for there's much that each of us can do once we're aware of these obstacles' existence and how they influence our lives and our deaths. So far, this book has explicated the first of them. The seven obstacles are:

1. Difficulty distinguishing among dying situations
2. Trouble determining when enough is enough
3. Over-reliance on advance directives
4. Exposure to medical snafus (misadventures and/or medical errors)
5. Ignorance regarding life-support matters including systemic overrides
6. Inability to advocate medically for a loved one or oneself
7. The Opaque Dying Marketplace

These obstacles grow from the personal to the situational to the environmental. The first and seventh obstacles are large: part of our cultural background, so big that we are affected by them even though we may not perceive them. Obstacles two through six begin with something deep inside us and get progressively larger and outward in scope. Recognizing each successive obstacle gets more challenging, and mitigating each successive obstacle requires more knowledge and skill.

These obstacles are practical in nature, the third leg of our end-of-life management tripod (the three legs being advance planning and proxy assignment; spiritual self-improvement; and practical knowledge, foresight, and skills). Unless we know that these obstacles exist, we may be taken entirely by surprise or overcome by shock when we encounter them—and we are likely to be ineffective in dealing with them. Unless we understand why and how the obstacles arise and function, we are unlikely to be able to forecast them, to quickly act to sidestep them, or to mitigate their damage after we've become ensnared. At its worst, ensnarement means that patient-families will traverse their dying territory under the influence of mainstream medicine's defaults and our own insistence on death denial, leading directly toward extended treatments and overmedicalized dying in the harder Matrix landings.

The obstacles tend to be linked. When one arises, it's likely that others have arisen also or will shortly arise. To help envision this and underscore that obstacles to peaceful dying arise together, here are two analogies.

The first analogy is the clock—specifically, what's known as the movement, the mechanism that moves the hands. In non-digital timepieces, that means gears. Gears, wheels with interlocking teeth, turn together. When one moves, all move. Left as set, they move slowly; the seconds, minutes, and hours tick by—as do the weeks, months, and years of long declines. When we adjust the time, we pull out a pin and spin the gears rapidly, zipping through hours and minutes with a single swipe of a finger, the timepiece hands inextricably linked—akin to the rapid pace of medical crises and the nature of obstacles to peaceful dying. Whether moving slowly or quickly, end-of-life obstacles tend to gear up together.

The second analogy is the train. Obstacles are sequenced, at first pulling, then eventually pushing us along. When dire events occur, some momentum evidences itself. The longer the obstacle train becomes (e.g., the more obstacles we experience) the greater the overall momentum becomes—for this discussion, momentum toward some outcome we have said or promised that we didn't want to experience.

Let's now examine each of the seven obstacles to dying in peace comprising To Die in Peace: Our Rights of Passage.

Obstacle 1:
Difficulty Distinguishing Among Dying Situations

> **Obstacle** Oversimplifying imagined late-life and dying scenarios increases our vulnerability to experiencing exactly those dying situations that we say we want to avoid.
>
> **Solution** Identifying and naming the full range of dying situations helps us to see our end days as traversing a dying territory, with way stations and landings that we can aim for or aim away from. Naming all our dying situations may stimulate us to take additional steps, beyond directives and spiritual engagement, to manage and mitigate everyday obstacles to dying in peace.

If you've arrived here by reading sequentially through this book devoted to examining this obstacle, you've seen that we tend to oversimplify when imagining where and how we die, usually limiting our thinking to two opposites. The first, usually and often deservedly viewed as tragic, is the ICU. The second, presumably wonderful for all, is at home. We fail to recognize that many other distinctly different dying situations exist, let alone distinguish among them. This blindness serves as a backdrop against which we try to grope our way toward, then through, our dying time.

Windrum's Matrix of Dying Terms identifies and distinguishes between 17 dying situations that comprise our dying territory. The Matrix provides new language with which we can identify every dying situation in our time and culture. Understanding our dying territory as a place with distinct way stations and destinations ("landings"), we become newly oriented. If you're like me, you may then wonder how you can get from where you are now to where you'd prefer to die within our dying territory—and how to avoid landing in dying situations that you would prefer to avoid.

Whenever the topic of dying arises, most of us express how

we *don't* want to die. How many of us have practical knowledge to ensure that we don't? How do we develop a sense of how to increase our likelihood of dying peacefully according to our preferred vision? Obstacles two through seven in To Die at Peace: Our Rights of Passage provide us with a framework to achieve that goal. For some obstacles, the explanations and examples are sufficient in and of themselves as solutions to the problems they address. Solving other obstacles will require an additional investment of time and study in order to position us to act, in advance and in the moment, to mitigate their ill effects. (Obstacles two through six represent issues addressed in *Notes from the Waiting Room*, newly restated.)

Obstacle 2:
Trouble Determining When enough is Enough

> **Obstacle** Because we can't answer the question, "When is enough enough?" we tend to re-engage in extreme medical treatments at ages and stages of decline beyond which those treatments are helpful (and which could be harmful). Doing so leads us toward harder dying, the kinds of deaths we say we wish to avoid.
>
> **Solution** By acknowledging our prior medical engagement as heroic, we give ourselves a frame of reference with which to evaluate whether or not the amount of medically heroic action we have previously taken adds up to "enough." Doing so may provide us the strength to decline risky treatments that could leave us worse off than we already are or, conversely, provide the certainty that we're ready to proceed with the treatment being considered.

I remember sitting around the kitchen table with my sister and parents, who by their 80s had had numerous life-enhancing and several lifesaving engagements with medicine. Like many elders and adult children, we had no answers when pondering the wisdom or danger of future medical treatments. My mother used to ask, "When is enough enough?" At that time, asked in the abstract, none of us could answer. After experiencing both of my parents' terminal hospitalizations, I learned to place the question in an answerable context. That context is heroicism. Heroicism is a lesser form of heroism and I use the former intentionally. Heroics are larger than life, the stuff of gods and immortals. Heroicism is something we mortals can and do engage in. And the answer to "When is enough enough?" may be found by answering "How many medically heroic actions have I engaged in? Have I done enough to extend or save my life, enough times, to assess that what I've done thus far is enough?" In other words, when does our very human heroicism morph into an attempt at immortal-scale heroics?

My father's medical trajectory provided me the context. His first life-and-death engagement with medicine, his first instance of heroicism, occurred 19 years before his death, with his first of two double cardiac bypass operations. His heart attack, resuscitation by electroshock (which I witnessed), and surgery occurred without his input. That medicine saved him and countless like him is a testament to our times' miracles, and we are grateful.

Dad was 65 years old at the time. Medicine provided him and our family two decades more time. My family did not have this timeframe in mind during Dad's last weeks—or before them, or we might have dug deeper into the pacemaker testing to assess its risks. During his medically enabled extra decades, Dad underwent a second double bypass (bad on him for not embracing lifestyle changes which might have precluded the need for it!); endured a failed and then a repeat hip replacement surgery; and subscribed to ongoing pharmaceutical management of high blood pressure, diabetes, unpleasant conditions related to bypass surgery such as fluid retention, and severely reduced cardiac function. I came to view these as heroic actions and to see that Mort's period of medical heroicism had begun with his first heart attack in 1985.

As I write this, I am now 65 years of age. Unlike my father, I am in good health; a few emergent experiences that raise questions, but no disease or serious conditions, and I ingest exactly zero prescription medications. But like my father, I have entered what is statistically the last quarter of my life. In fact, I've been there for the past five years, as has any American 60 or over. I don't like framing my age this way but death-literacy requires that I do, because I'm nearing the age that anything can, and may, happen to me. Because I'm healthy I don't dwell on dying (an ironic admission, I know...), but I've long said that from 70 years out there ought to be no surprises for any of us should we or a loved one suffer a serious or fatal health setback. OK, that's a bit of an oversimplification but, statistically, we may succumb anytime during the last eighth of our lives.

And what of the iconic, hail-Mary attempts to stave off death during some heroic hospitalization? In a state similar to the one I was in when I received the "zillion words for snow" message that led to Windrum's Matrix of Dying Terms, I once calculated that at 84 years of age my father's approximately three-week terminal hospitalization represented 7/10,000 of his lifespan. 7/10,000! Such a minuscule amount yet so full of life, love and heartbreak. Must it always come down to our last 7/10,000? When is the nature of our last 7/10,000 of our lifespan formulated? Do we, must we, always crave more time?

Through his years of hospice rounds, the Canadian end-of-life activist Stephen Jenkinson, in his book *Die Wise*, identifies what he calls "More Time" as a core factor motivating people who struggle against impending death. Extending his observation to my lexicon, we engage in medical heroicism in order to get more More Time to live. In our hunger for More Time we misconstrue when our More Time actually is granted. Most of us view More Time as time obtained in the present for the future; time obtained like a rabbit pulled out of a magician's hat, where the doctors are magicians and the hat is full of advanced medical procedures that prevent dying. While frequently true, we forget the times that we've already lived through fraught medical circumstances and have already been granted considerable lengths of More Time. We forget that yesterday's gift of future time is today's now and that *yesterday's More Time, previously granted, has been lived*. I propose that, for many of us with complicated medical histories, our More Time may lie behind us; that we have already been granted it and have already lived it. Without the viewpoint provided by assessing prior medical engagement, we don't realize that we've been granted and lived More Time, so we can't answer that universal question, "When is enough enough?" If we've accounted for our prior medical engagement, we can better answer that question, each for ourselves. It's possible we'll say, "enough is enough" and it's possible we'll say, "I haven't had enough quite yet." At least we'll have a coherent frame of reference.

With 20/20 hindsight, I can only wonder if my family's approach to our desires for Dad's final years might have changed had we been able to frame them by assessing how much medical heroism Dad had already manifested throughout the last quarter of his life. Making this assessment is crucial because of the obstacles that medical heroism exposes us to. Before we examine them, we need to identify and ponder one other obstacle, one that works hand-in-hand with our willingness to act heroically that one more time...

Obstacle 3:
Over-reliance on Advance Directives

> <u>Obstacle</u> Our assumption that the advance directives we've executed provide an ironclad or guaranteed peaceful

dying experience tends to make us feel complacent, fully protected. We therefore are disinclined to invest the time and effort required to educate ourselves about many other end-of-life obstacles to dying in peace.

Solution By recognizing that advance directives are neither ironclad nor guarantees, but rather a necessary yet loosely woven "safety net," we see our directives as the first of many steps to take to protect ourselves against the types of late-life and dying experiences we say we want to avoid.

Because we are told so many times from so many sources that we ought to, even *must*, create advance directives, we tend to think that they will be 100% protective and effective. The documents are, in fact, challenging—requiring us to grapple with matters we would prefer not to, and to engage in deep self-reflection to prepare. Surely something so weighty must be very powerful.

They can be. They ought to be. Ultimately, they may be. There's no guarantee that they will take effect quickly because between your directives and your peaceful demise are a batch of circumstances, a range of dying situations, a host of medical professionals and entities, and family members and loved ones, all co-mingling as a demise unfolds over time. Things happen—hopefully informed by and channeled by directives. But often this is not the case; then we pull out the directives to try to undo things that have already occurred. Our directives become a fallback used retrospectively rather than a roadmap used proactively. Having been in such situations twice for a period totaling about five weeks, I learned that directives in and of themselves do not prevent any one of us from experiencing an onslaught of treatments over time that preclude peaceful dying, especially if we have assumed that we can rely on directives alone.

The core advance directives are:

- A durable medical power of attorney naming our surrogate decision-makers should we become incapacitated, giving them legal and recognized authority to speak for us and to direct our medical treatments on our behalf. This will require them to skillfully act as our surrogate
- A Living Will stating what medical treatments and life supports we do or don't want to accept, ideally including some discussion of our values and baselines for what makes life worthwhile to us.
- A Do Not Resuscitate Order (DNR), which, unlike the other two, is a doctor's order and must be made in consultation with one's doctor and signed by them.

These three directives are the basics. We might consider adding a POLST or MOST form (Physician's Orders for Life-Sustaining Treatment or Medical Orders for Scope of Treatment), which list a range of specific life-support interventions in a checkbox format that's both more comprehensive than a DNR and easier for first responders to quickly assess. As with the DNR, a POLST/MOST must be executed in consultation with and signed by one's doctor. Other more specialized directives exist, for example, limiting transport to some place or directing transport away from some place—like Do Not Transport for those in nursing facilities who want to stipulate that they not be transported to a hospital should their condition deteriorate, and a sectarian or "get me out of here" directive should you find yourself inadvertently hospitalized in a facility with religious strictures limiting one's full range of end-of-life choice. Other directives exist; I describe them in Appendix C.

Directives do not guarantee outcomes. As I stated early in this book, advance directives seem to me to be either presented as or misunderstood to be guarantors of peaceful dying, as if they come with an implied promise governing the conformance of any medical professional to whom we present them. Directives might perform to perfection if circumstances play out nicely. Or they might

not. A range of variables can render our directives moot, including:
- When directives cannot be located by first responders (I know of one elderly couple who refuse to post them on their refrigerator, the primary location that emergency responders look for them, because the envelope reminds them of their mortality).
- When directives cannot be found or produced by their owners at the moment of need (although one set ought to reside in your bank's safe deposit box, it's useless there except as a master from which to make copies—copies needed on your fridge, in your freezer, on your person, in all your vehicles, and in the easily retrievable possession of all your named surrogate(s), perhaps even all your family members).
- When directives are not logged into a patient's medical chart during institutionalization or hospitalizations—an elderly couple could forget to present a copy of their directives upon admission, or the documents might get lost between the admissions desk and the unit where a loved one is bedded.
- When directives do not accompany a person during transit from one facility to another.
- When directives are ignored or overridden by oneself, by surrogates, or by medical personnel from first responders to facilities and surgeons (Obstacle 5 discusses overrides to our directives).

Obstacles 1–3 Reflection

In the opening section of this chapter, I mentioned that obstacles to dying in peace usually arise together. Considering the first three obstacles to peaceful dying, we already have the makings of a clockwork mechanism, a train of decisions that can pull us away from the dying experience we say we want and push us into situations we say we don't want:

1. Our failure to distinguish between dying situations leaves us without a useful organizing concept for the situations within which

we die, unaware of way stations throughout our dying territory and without a map for navigating. We literally don't know with any specificity what may be in front of us; all we have are vague fears of protracted dying in the ICU offset by vague thoughts of dying at home as a panacea, whether or not we've considered our caregiving and medical needs or soberly assessed our support networks.

2. Without a framework to evaluate our history of medical engagement, when we need to answer the question, "When is enough enough?", we may be inclined to say, "Well, not yet," and tend to try and try again. We engage in repeat medical treatments at later and later ages and at greater and greater risk. Medicine, to its discredit, generally fails to disclose such risks, and we, to our discredit, generally don't want to know about them.

3. We might feel safe going down this path because we've assumed, been told, or believe an implied promise that our advance directives will protect us from the types of circumstances and dying situations we have declared that we want to avoid. Thus, we may feel safer pursuing medical treatments than prudence might suggest. We may do so without knowing of or understanding the primary risks that accompany late-life medical treatments. We might do so despite having prior experience with the types of deaths we say we want to avoid.

Before proceeding, a question: If you've already experienced a loved one's peace-less dying, does any of this feel familiar? It does to me. When I asked myself, regarding my parents' deaths, "Why did we fail to achieve peaceful deaths?", all of this, all these thoughts arose over time in answer.

Where the first three obstacles address circumstances leading to medical engagement, the next three obstacles identify troubles encountered as a result of medical engagement. Obstacles 4 and 5 encapsulate these risks. Obstacle 6 identifies a major requisite skill for managing them that virtually every one of us lacks.

Obstacle 4:
Exposure to Medical Snafus (Misadventures and/or Medical Errors)

Obstacle Late-life medical treatments carry an increased risk of destabilization. Misadventure (undergoing a dubiously chosen or unnecessary test or procedure) can introduce or accelerate decline, sometimes severely. Medical error can debilitate and kill. Sometimes, misadventure results in situations that are more prone to medical error; the two snafus are linked. Medicine downplays and under-discloses these risks.

Solution Knowing that misadventure and error are distinctly possible may stimulate us to more carefully assess late-life medical treatments.

Misadventure* is defined as a reversal of fortune. Consider my father's experience, the severe breakdown of his stable state. His condition prior to the cardiac pacemaker eligibility test was stable, albeit limited. As an example, medicines for his heart troubles resulted in fluid buildup, hence the need to take diuretic pills twice a day. Because he relied on a walker (and a scooter) he needed to stay home, in close proximity to the toilet, for up to five hours after taking the diuretic—every morning and every evening. However, between those periods he was fully functional and independent, out and about in the world every day during his afternoon time. The nuclear pacemaker testing he chose to undergo, where traceable dye added to the bloodstream enters a

---

* Thanks to end-of-life author Katy Butler for suggesting the use of "misadventure" when discussing medical snafus.

chemically extra-stimulated heart, broke his stability; he was not hardy enough to withstand the stress. In other words, the procedure was too risky for his condition. His medical "crash" landed him in a hospital bed, susceptible to the risks of late-life hospitalization. Medical misadventure—misjudging the risks of invasive testing while desirous of the potential benefits—landed Dad in-hospital. Medical error occurred, and more misadventure ensued as he lay there.

Medical error is the third leading cause of death in the United States after heart failure and cancer and before every other cause of death, whether disease or accident. Medicine barely acknowledges this. We won't find medical error listed in "Top Ten Causes of Death" charts ritually published in major medical journals (see the *Journal of Participatory Medicine* article "It's Time to Account for Medical Error in 'Top Ten Causes of Death Charts'"—Google "Windrum JoPM" to find it). In my father's case he, and by extension the family, suffered medical error—the hospital-caused MRSA bloodstream infection from which he died. His death certificate listed cardiac failure as the cause of death rather than medical error (of course his heart failed, we stopped his various life-supporting heart medications when he entered hospice). The practice of fudging causes of death adds insult to harm and compounds end-of-life problems by limiting our ability—personally and societally—to assess risk.

An additional risk of hospitalization at advanced age is hospital-caused delirium—the loss of mental stability brought on by the stress of severe illness, exacerbated by typical hospital environments. Triggers include infection, pain, adverse effects of medications (so-called "side" effects), isolation, and a disruptive environment. Hospital delirium is more than a passing condition; one gets worse for having it. Delirium accelerates decline. During the weeks between acquiring MRSA and entering hospice, as Dad lay hospitalized, he exhibited well-known symptoms of delirium: disorientation, altered mental states, and hallucinations. The staff didn't observe it; I did. I didn't recognize or understand it in 2005. It was another contributing factor to our angst.

All of this represents the antithesis of peaceful dying. We rolled the dice—and lost.

Obstacle 5:
Ignorance Regarding Life-support Matters Including Systemic Overrides

> **Obstacle** Our directives and preferences limiting life-support treatments may be disregarded in various medical service settings from the street to the surgical suite—placing us at risk of landing in very extreme situations that we wished to avoid. We do not expect or foresee these outcomes because we don't know about them until they happen to us.
>
> **Solution** Understanding how various medical personnel approach their work—their workplace rules, default positions, and values—will prepare us to engage with them in advance of and during dire circumstances. Understanding that overrides to our directives may occur prepares us to advocate effectively.

We are grateful, perhaps in awe, when life-support technology saves a life on the street. We appreciate, with wonder, when life support sustains us through now-routine surgeries. We tend to recoil at the thought of life supports as instruments of futile, endless late-life medical treatment that may become torturous.

The application of life-support technologies is a complex aspect of modern medicine. It began in the mid-twentieth century with the introduction of the cardiac defibrillator, followed by ventilators (breathing machines). These advances led to the modern ICU, electronic implants like cardiac pacemakers, and portable life-support equipment deployed with first responders and located in business settings and public buildings. Life-support equipment is now everywhere. Both our society and medical systems are oriented toward using it regardless of a person's age and condition, although resuscitation is "successful" at best only about 15% of the time it is used on the elderly ill. "Success" means only that recipients didn't die. However, they will usually be much worse off after resuscitation than they were before it.

The systemic default position for treating people with life-support equipment shows up in institutional policies, personal and medical professional inclinations, surprise overrides to advance directives, and even the verbal directives of surrogates representing critically ill patients with directives limiting life supports.

Policies, inclinations, and overrides promoting rapid life-support deployment constitute a strong current; it's the way things flow. Anyone who doesn't want to swim with this current will necessarily have to swim against it.

When might we want to swim against the life-support current? To draw on the solution to Obstacle 2 to peaceful dying—trouble determining when enough is enough—when we've decided that enough is enough. Even so, any of us might change our minds when the abstract becomes real, when we or a loved one actually face the possibility of dying—in which case enough wasn't really enough. Know that the life-support current is strong, so if you are sure that enough is enough, be prepared to dig in your heels and apply your advocate skills against what could be a forceful effort to persuade you otherwise. That effort has been known to include false hope, guilt-tripping, and shame. Know, too, that once deployed, life supports can be very hard to remove; the current is still flowing, and now you, as a medical proxy, may wonder if by ordering their removal you would be directly responsible for a loved one's death (in most cases not). I know this conundrum well, having personally wrestled with it indirectly during my mother's demise, and directly as my father's proxy during his Erroneous terminal hospitalization.

Three streams feed the life-support current. Let's navigate each one.

Life-support Current, Stream 1:
Institutional Life-support Policies

Institutions have policies. Policies that impact the public ought to be public (not all are, see Obstacle 7 below). For statements by "brick and mortar" institutions expressing their policies, look on walls and columns in waiting rooms, in brochures set on counters in clinics or admission areas, and in binders or other printed materials in inpatient rooms. For mobile institutions, e.g., first responders (ambulance services and fire and police departments), their policy is to apply life-support methods and equipment to prevent deaths. Emergency rooms are similar: the goal is to save a life, stabilize a patient, and move them to a bed in a ward or the ICU where their condition and status may then be sorted out. If you don't want to undergo forceful resuscitation, the ER is not a place you want to visit.

Life-support Current, Stream 2:
Professional Inclinations

Powerful inclinations toward lifesaving emanate from the civilian and professional worlds. Since most of us have not really engaged in end-of-life planning (as you know by now, I do not consider conversations and directives as constituting advance planning), we are inclined to accept heroic treatment even if we have said "enough is enough." Humanity's life force is a powerful drive; what's different for us compared to our ancestors is that modern medicine is so effective at extending existence. We civilians cling to hope, and medical professionals are loath to dash it. Medicine's mission is built upon bolstering hope, not extinguishing it. The inclination of medical professionals to save first and sort out the patient's status afterward is bred deeply throughout medical school, during internships, and in everyday medical practice. They're trained to err on the side of caution; allowing someone to die without engaging in every technologically possible heroic measure is believed to equate to doing harm (ironically, many such measures actually cause harm). Also operating behind the scenes are business considerations—when and where people die can affect both surgeon success/failure ratings and hospital facility ratings. The U.S. government financially penalizes hospitals that fail to meet certain benchmarks. And the longer people remain patients the longer payers can be billed for medical services.

We all are in this current together. Sometimes it moves slowly, often it moves rapidly with decisions required in the moment; always it is strong.

Life-support Current, Stream 3:
Overrides to Our Anti-Resuscitation Directives

Overrides to our advance directives are the deeper currents in my experience, often hidden and destabilizing to patient-families who may suddenly find themselves caught by an unexpected override. The expectation is that our living wills, DNRs, and POLSTs ought to protect us! Well, they may or may not, depending upon whether the forms are present at the necessary moment and whether their wording is precise and limiting or vague and open-ended. In any case, there are situations in which medicine claims the right to override our directives. Surgery, especially when performed in the operating theater, is the primary situation where a profound difference in values may inform the orientation of civilians versus doctors and facilities.

Medicine claims priority and authority over directives against life support during surgery and for various lengths of time after surgery, during which our DNRs and POLSTs are moot, overridden. If our heart or breathing stops while we're on the table, "code" will be called, we will be resuscitated and the life supports will remain in place post-op. The trouble is that most of us don't know this, we assume that our directives will accompany us into the surgical suite. During my father's demise we didn't learn of this until very nearly the time of the surgery to drain his MRSA-infected wrist. The override was a deal breaker. Dad bailed; this was the moment that enough was enough. The issue could have been introduced and brokered one or several days before the juncture, rather than being sprung on us at that late moment in our crucible. The timing only added to our sense of shock and our experience of harm. It's possible to try to learn in advance if the doctors you'll be partnering with and the facilities housing you will override directives during surgery or not. I'll address this below in our discussion of Obstacles 6 and 7.

The solution to Obstacle 5, ignorance regarding life-support matters including systemic overrides, is threefold: know that policies, inclinations, and insistence on overrides exist; always expect life-support measures to be applied every time, everywhere; learn what to do about overrides, i.e. how to advocate effectively in medical situations.

Obstacle 6:
Inability to Advocate Medically for a Loved One or Oneself

> **Obstacle** Knowing how to advocate in medical situations is a learned skill, outside the bounds of advance directives and spiritual engagement. Because almost no training is available, our knowledge of issues, problems, and solutions, and our skill as an advocate is usually obtained by experience, much of which is bitter. We learn under duress, at our most vulnerable, and in response to risks, danger, and harm.
> **Solution** We may increase our readiness by engaging in independent study; finding and reading books; attending live trainings; and joining online membership groups and

discussion forums. These resources offer guidance based on individuals' prior real-world experiences (I list the best in Appendix C.) Forewarned and sensitized, we may learn to anticipate and respond rather than merely react. Ultimately, increasing our advocacy skills requires experience—there are few role-play substitutes.

Medicine tells us to assign trusted others to assist in directing our medical affairs, and to represent us should we become unable to speak for ourselves. Medicine tells us to come prepared to take an active part in our medical experiences, seeking treatments we want and acting to protect ourselves against treatments we don't want. Medicine's instruction acknowledges how important this is. Have you noticed that medicine doesn't really tell us why this is important... let alone how to do it, or to go about learning?

To be fair, some information is provided. Brochures and inpatient binder inserts offer some guidance. That guidance will be thin compared to what we must know; the topic is thick, the task huge. And for serious or long medical engagements, advocacy requires a personal team working in shifts.

Reflect on the preceding obstacles: anti-resuscitation overrides, medical misadventures and medical error, over-reliance on directives, unexamined heroism, and inadequately distinguishing among dying situations. Learning how to advocate medically is a major effort. It's bigger than any of us want and deeper than most of us have the time and energy to do. And for most of our lives, in most instances, medicine works splendidly; when things go right, our advocacy chops are neither tested nor needed. Yet we must hone them and apply them during any medical engagement, for we never know when things may go wrong. And the nearer we get to the end of our lives, the more the balance between safety and risk changes, for a range of reasons. (The reasons become evident through reading books on how to approach the end of life, what to expect, and how to advocate; and by reflecting on demises we may already have experienced.)

How do we learn to advocate medically? The best way is by studying a growing body of literature. I offer "best of the best" lists in Appendix C, at the end of *Notes from the Waiting Room: Managing a Loved One's End-of-Life Hospitalization* and at AxiomAction.com/bibliography, and within some posts at AxiomAction.com/blog. I highly recommend joining the Facebook group Slow Medicine for the guidance, wisdom, and even compassion offered there by medical professionals, activists, and lay people. Seek live workshops if you can find them, but know that workshops on how to advocate medically are not exactly in demand. I offer To Die in Peace: Our Rights of Passage workshops on an occasional basis. Do not expect events like panel discussions to offer much, if anything, regarding in-depth aspects of advocating medically. In my experience, both the makeup and discussion engaged in by end-of-life panels hasn't materially changed over the course of my involvement in this work; I have found both extremely lacking.

At the end, we will find our landing—or some landing will claim us. Today, implied and self-generated promises may shape our expectations of how dying will unfold. Learning how to advocate medically will play a major role in how well we uphold the promises we take to heart and the promises we make.

Obstacles 4–6 Reflection

Where Obstacles 1–3 present as non-specific internal and external impediments (we can't articulate our preferred dying situations; we have trouble identifying when enough is enough; we are lulled into a false sense of security by the idea that advance directives will fully protect us), obstacles 4–6 are specific to medical events that we might experience. For instance:

• A loved one may crash medically, undergoing immediate and significant degradation that would not have occurred had we known the risks of some proposed or urged course of treatment and opted out.

• We might experience shock and harm when our directives or instructions prohibiting life-support treatments are overridden with zero or little notice, placing our patient-family in extreme circumstances that in themselves may jerk us into a landing that we wanted to avoid.

• A bitter demise of a patient-family member might teach us that had we acquired the knowledge and skill to advocate medically, we might have been able to foresee and influence or negotiate an outcome better aligned with our values and desires.

To the extent we are unaware that these obstacles exist, they will take us by surprise—e.g., we will feel shocked. If we are unable to forecast and mitigate one or more obstacles, if we are unskilled or unable to mitigate the obstacles' effects before negative outcomes occur, our patient-family will experience the harm of entrapment in situations that we do not want to experience—typically some kind of protracted death in machine-controlled environments. When adverse circumstances occur that could have been avoided with foresight and prior knowledge, we may experience the extrinsic pain that results from unnecessary harm. If these results happen to us despite promises we've accepted or made, we may experience a new, additional pain: promise pain.

Shock and harm, and extrinsic and promise pain associated with the end-of-life interrupt, interfere with, and even prevent dying *in* peace. With enough interference, patient-families will likely not experience a death *at* peace, either.

A final obstacle exists as a backdrop to the other obstacles, one so amorphous that we don't realize it's there. I've become sensitized to it throughout enough years and inquiries I've made of medicine to sense a pattern. I've named it the Opaque Dying Marketplace.

Obstacle 7:
The Opaque Dying Marketplace

> **Obstacle**   When we ask probing, specific questions to try to learn about end-of-life services provided by individuals and systems, especially in advance of any particular need, medical professionals may offer only vague answers or may refuse to answer at all.
>
> **Solution**   Becoming aware that evasion in response to legitimate questions represents a pattern can stimulate our resolve to push for the answers we seek and deserve.

Advance planning can be viewed as our personal and group disclosure to medicine. Medicine's consistent and unified guidance to engage in advance planning, including directives, presents a powerful front. The acknowledged value of advance planning aside, medicine asks and almost demands that we arrive ready to answer questions about end-of-life matters—which medical treatments we will and will not accept, under which circumstances.

For those who have taken medicine's guidance to heart it follows that, over time, a population will begin to generate questions. Any serious person looking ahead to end-of-life situations, especially if previously harmed by adverse end-of-life experiences, is bound to produce questions in advance of repeat engagement.

If you're like me, you may sit back with a suite of advance directives and memories of prior deaths gone badly and muse about yours or a loved one's future. You may project your thoughts toward situations that your documents are intended to influence and your memories induce you to feel wary of. You may wonder, "how do I trust all what I must trust? Might it better serve me and my loved ones were I to ask medicine the questions arising in my mind now, before we find ourselves in the thick of the next demise in our family?"

This matters a lot when we want to identify medical professionals and facilities who share our end-of-life values and orientation, to minimize the risk of ending up in a haphazardly forced end-of-life marriage where values clash in dire circumstances with little or no time to find new partners.

The idea of doctors and patients as partners is not new. In medical reform circles its necessity is promoted and its absence is decried. My idea of partnership is that each entity brings their own knowledge to the partnership and that each party is fundamentally equal. In particular for this discussion, equal to ask and have meaningfully answered questions about end-of-life matters in any setting and at any time. Especially when the questions are posed by people who will one day be patients and surrogate decision makers.

If our advance directives equate to our disclosure, does medicine reciprocate? How willing is medicine—each doctor and every facility—to disclose its orientation as providers of end-of-life treatments far enough in advance that we may factor their answers into our advance planning?

Here's what I've learned from my periodic attempts between 2005 and 2017 to ask medicine for answers: medicine will talk on its terms according to its timing, not ours. Medicine will exert control and place conditions on the types of conversations it will engage in with civilians, including when it will engage. Under those conditions, medicine may talk face to face to you about you, and to me about me, but not to us about itself, and not unless you or I have a presenting medical need.

This is a troubling observation. Obviously, my own experiences represent a small sample set, but as you'll read below, I go further than most people would in posing advance end-of-life questions. I've ended up feeling frustrated, distrustful, and annoyed. After all, I've taken the guidance to plan in advance to heart. I've realized that family conversations and legal forms go only so far. I'm left with questions—not about my condition (I'm thankfully healthy as I write this), but rather about how the doctors and facilities I'm considering as partners approach their provision of late-life medical services. How long, how far into my own lifetime, must I wait in order to have the questions answered? It doesn't matter whether the failure is systemic (the circular situation of a policy preventing the disclosure of policies) or situational (an individual or business unable or unwilling to make a statement, or that makes a denial without explanation). For all of us, what effect does medicine's silence have on our quest to die in, and at, peace?

In the best of circumstances, interactions at the end of life become relationships... personal, heartfelt, humane, perhaps transcendent. Before getting there, interactions are exploratory, essentially transactional. When our ability to learn (let alone choose) is stymied because medicine fails or refuses to answer basic questions before we get entangled in some personal medical emergency, I feel logically impelled to name that condition. I've named it the *Opaque Dying Marketplace* (in Latin, the language of medicine: *Opacum Emporium Mortis*.)

This is unsettling, as is knowing that some in medicine have a hard time accepting this framing. To quote the Never Say Die Rap, "I don't mean to be mean." Many good women and men work in medicine. Framing civilian interaction with medical professionals in commercial terms may offend. It need not if we consider the following.

Describing a widespread condition is not a personal indictment. Learning how to advocate medically requires someone to translate the language and prerogatives of medicine into civilian experience. My role is to examine, reveal, and describe the layperson's experience and to suggest ways to mitigate ill effects. As I asked in my TEDx talk, To Die in Peace: New Terms of Engagement: Why do we fail to die in peace? Who owns our dying? Who controls? What is required of you, and of me, to die in peace?

Unfortunately, too many medical professionals endure stressful working conditions including short appointments, byzantine electronic systems, punitive financial costs, and other modern workplace pressures. My heart goes out to people so afflicted, yet I cannot fix those and am unqualified to address them.

I am aware of doctors and nurses dedicated to improving medicine and our interaction with it. People like the late geriatrician Dennis McCullough who, in his highly informative book, *My Mother, Your Mother: Embracing Slow Medicine*, gifts us by describing our declining days as stages we can anticipate. Or the surgeon Atul Gawande who, in *Being Mortal*, distinguishes between safety and autonomy to frame this most significant late-life conundrum. And Dr. Bernard Lown's Lown Institute and its Right Care initiative focused on solving both endemic overtreatment and undertreatment. Even taken together these additions to our understanding, and more like them, do not add up to systemic change; the Opaque Dying Marketplace endures as a meta-level condition.

Lastly, we must recognize the proper ordering of engagement. The personal relationships civilians and medical professionals hope for, the ones that offer possibilities for higher meaning, do not come first. To have those experiences we must first find one another. In the free market that means providing meaningful descriptions and indicators. Even highly trained people exist as agents in a marketplace; facilities and institutions most definitely, dispassionately do. For civilians inclined to plan ahead, the relationships come after we've navigated the marketplace.

― ―

The Opaque Dying Marketplace is broad, a meta-level obstacle existing as a backdrop to the other obstacles and affecting our experience of all of them. Like the air around us, the Opaque Dying Marketplace applies pressure. We don't realize it because it's always there.

We encounter and consciously feel the *Opacum Emporium Mortis* when we seek information about end-of-life matters in advance of an acute need and are met with vague answers or no answers at all. Although people in the medical system may rationalize why they fail to honestly and transparently answer questions, our questions, despite deep implications, are straightforward and answers ought to be forthcoming.

Having had severe experiences during my parents' hospitalized demises, I now have questions to which I would like answers. My experience in getting answers is mixed and troubling. Without answers, we're adrift; we can't make informed advance decisions. (For instance, if area hospitals differ in the policies governing the interplay between anti-resuscitation directives and their overrides, which hospital would you prefer to be in if you can arrange to have a choice? Which doctor might you like to build a relationship with given your values and desires around late-life health matters and dying?) A few basic descriptions of doctor and institutional orientation around several key aspects affecting late life and the end of life could be easily communicated.

I'll preface a discussion of the Opaque Dying Marketplace with a story from my childhood in suburban New York from which I'll draw an analogy about disclosure. It's slightly risqué, so if you take offense easily, be forewarned.

Those days, circa 1960 and second grade, our street, Janos Lane in West Hempstead, New York, was busy after school and after dinner with lots of children out playing. My immediate neighbors were a family with two kids, Johnny and Mary. Janos Lane curved around a lot-sized pond nestled below grade. We avoided it in warm weather but during winter we all sledded down onto the pond and skated atop it. The pond drained through a culvert that ran below the street. One day, Johnny and Mary approached me to play "I'll show you mine if you show me yours"—a game of childhood sexual exploration wherein participants expose themselves in turn for the curious other to see, perhaps for the first time. We found a quiet time and entered the culvert. Mary and I were to exchange revelations; Johnny held the flashlight. I went first, lit bright by Johnny's light. After recomposing myself I said, "Your turn, Mary" whereupon Johnny yelled "Run, Mary!" Run they did. I had shown Mary mine; she did not show me hers.

The youthful exploratory game relied upon a quid pro quo—I'll show you mine and you show me yours. We were young and silly, yet the showing regarded intimate matters. Today, we grownups want mature engagement regarding intimate matters affecting the most sacred future time of our lives. Ironically, it's childish of medicine to run, to hide, to refuse. Only this time, it's not a game.

The initial transactions around end-of-life matters require equality to develop into trusting relationships. The absence of reciprocity is an abrogation of responsibility and perpetuates death illiteracy. Medicine knows that directive documents are tenuous at best and can fail for various reasons. I find it extraordinarily hypocritical that medicine refuses to answer basic end-of-life questions—in advance of acute personal need—after exhorting us to answer its questions via our advance directives *under the rubric of advance planning.*

Have you asked medicine to "show theirs" to you? Have they? I have asked—over a 12-year period, in Florida and in Colorado. Medicine has not shown me theirs. I'll cite four instances. The first was deadly, the second stymies informed choice, and the third and fourth stonewall citizens who take advance planning and peaceful dying to heart.

Opaque Dying Marketplace example, 2005:
Neither Advised of Nor Offered a Time-Based Trial

My first experience of medicine refusing to show us theirs was during my father's demise. It was passive, built into the system. I've cited Mort's story earlier in this book as an example of one end-of-life landing; here we'll delve into what turned out to be the ethical and existential crux we encountered and failed to deal with adequately, because we lacked the knowledge and skill to advocate effectively.

By age 84 Dad had been successfully managing a litany of serious conditions, most of them comorbidities: his heart was pumping at only one-third capacity due to two prior double bypasses, and he suffered from high blood pressure, diabetes, and the semi-crippling results of a failed hip replacement which had to be redone using a different implant. He was impaired yet fully functional and mobile, living independently, of agile mind, completely competent. After Mom's death a year prior, Dad wanted to return to Mile-high Colorado where the air is thin, after eight years in retirement at sea-level Florida. It was presumed and possibly likely that such a move, if at all physically possible, would require the assistance of an implanted cardiac pacemaker. He 'crashed' medically during pacemaker eligibility testing that used radioactive dye and a heart stimulant injected into the bloodstream as an alternative to stressing the heart by running on a treadmill, which he was of course unable to do. He became a hospital inpatient, and acquired the superbug MRSA through a urinary catheter. (Catheter-induced, hospital-acquired infections have since been defined as a "never-event"—an event that ought never occur—by the Centers for Medicare and Medicaid (CMS); now hospitals where too many never-events happen may be financially penalized.) The infection coursed through his bloodstream, swelling his wrist, which quite painfully mushroomed in size. He was intermittently delirious, which could have been caused by the stress of the medical crash, or the infection, or the hospital environment, his accelerated decline brought about by any or all of these. To try to reverse this onslaught, surgery was scheduled to drain the infection at his wrist. The procedure would be palliative in any case, relieving the intense pain, perhaps restoring Dad's use of his dominant hand. Because of his compromised heart the doctors required that the operation be under general anesthesia in the OR; they deemed local anesthetic or a nerve block in a less formal operating environment as too risky. Dad, Judy and I concurred. Then we had sprung on us, via the surgical release form delivered only several hours before the surgery was to occur, that Dad's DNR order would be suspended during surgery—if his heart stopped during surgery they would resuscitate him. We all rejected that; Dad didn't want to risk landing intubated in an ICU, the way Mom had died during her multi-week demise 15 months earlier. The doctors wouldn't budge. As Dad's proxy I spoke with the anesthesiologist who happened to also be the head of his department. He would not change position and offered nothing more. Not knowing how to ask leading questions, I was at the end of my uninformed ability to advocate in a medical context. Ending the conversation with the anesthesiologist, I realized that I had to go back to Dad and deliver his death sentence, for he was clear that he would not subject himself to the risk of ending up like Mom did.

Completely opaque to us was that an option did exist. Granted, I wasn't a good enough proxy to ask the anesthesiologist, "Is there anything else we can consider or negotiate?" And I oughtn't have had to; I was not a dying expert, the doctors serving the southern United States seaboard full of elderly dying Floridians and their families were. The option we should have been offered was then and is now well-known. It's called a time-based trial or a time trial. We and the doctors would have negotiated a fixed time period post-op after which, if it turned out that Dad wound up on life supports, we would remove them, honoring Dad's rejection of late-life Machine control. I would have agreed, and I think Dad would have agreed too, both Judy and I having his back to ensure compliance. We didn't have that choice because we weren't offered it, and we were too inexperienced as medical proxies to know about it. (I first learned about time-based trials 18 months after Dad died, while researching *Notes from the Waiting Room*. I'll never forget the moment during a phone conversation with nurse-ethicist Diann Uustal, when she asked: "didn't anyone offer your family a time-based trial?" I paused and the silence lengthened as I processed this new phrase and the implications of what Diann had asked....)

Back to Dad: By that point, a week and a half into Dad's hospitalization, we were all traumatized and shocked. It would be years before I learned how to unpack this situation; that medicine defaults to lifesaving at any and all costs; that doctors do not want people dying during their surgeries; that hospitals do not want people dying in their operating rooms; that any hospitalization at advanced age is significantly more risky for elders because the environment can induce and accelerate debility; that medical and governmental treatment of cause of death data hides prevalent risks of late-life medical treatments; that proclaiming a facility or practice to be "patient centered" is meaningless unless real patient-centric policies are in place. Withholding consent forms until the last minute and withholding treatment parameters during life and death decision-making does not qualify as patient-centric, nor does hanging banners trumpeting the facility's latest Joint Commission accreditation. Non-disclosure is opacity.

I do not know if patient-centricity was a "thing" in 2005. It seems to have emerged as a focus of attention around 2010. I did not know in 2005, and do not know now, if doctors and hospitals purposefully delay the introduction of surgical release forms for inpatients or if their system simply failed to deliver them to patient-families with more lead time. I do know the effect that late delivery has on people who have yet to learn what obstacles to anticipate, what to ask, what to forecast, and how to interact with the medical system when hospitalized. Late release-form delivery destabilizes patients and proxies who read and take them seriously, who may want to negotiate or strike certain clauses.

Doctors and facilities may be negatively graded and judged by death-during-surgery statistics. In some, perhaps many cases, that's unfair to them. And until medicine forces its governing bodies or influences the U.S. federal government to refine the parameters applied to compiling end-of-life statistics, it remains unfair to civilians who may find their DNRs overridden.

Opaque Dying Marketplace example, 2014:
The White Wall of Medical Silence

It would be nine years and two more instances of denial to impress upon me the prevalence and impact of opacity. The next occurrence was not passive, it was quite deliberate.

This second instance of medical opacity is directly related to the first. As you may now imagine, how hospitals deal with honoring or suspending DNRs during surgery is profoundly important to me; a hospital that offers to honor patient DNRs during surgery would be a more favorable candidate for my business.

Imagine my piqued interest, even delight, when I learned in early September 2014 that a local hospital system was about to implement a policy change allowing DNRs to stand during surgery! "This was huge", I thought. "A sea change!" Exciting and liberating for people who believe that patients ought to have more say in this matter. I don't recall how I learned of this, but to verify it I called the hospital over several days, asking to be put in contact with, in turn, the patient representative, the chaplain(s), the risk manager, and then the manager of patient safety and quality. The patient representative indicated that no policy change existed. I kept calling, seeking verification, leaving voice messages. About three weeks later I received a call from the clinical manager for nursing services, who verified the policy change, set for December 2014, and that the change was widely known by those working in the chain's facilities.

This was such welcome news to me that I naively thought that it was newsworthy, that the system would issue a press release and that regional media would pick up the story. I didn't read or hear one. In early and mid-December 2014 I left voicemail for the systemwide marketing manager, whose contact I obtained from the system website. I subsequently received an email from a physician who was also a top-level system executive, to whom the marketing manager had forwarded my email. He wrote that they did not disclose hospital policy. In so doing he erected what's known as "the white wall of silence": doctors' refusal to share information (white refers to doctors' white coats). I didn't bother writing back.

This is as opaque as things can get regarding an issue about which people who have made advance directives are rightfully interested. We would like to learn more about medical arrangements available in our own communities, to better prepare ourselves for the day when we must make such important medical choices. We deserve to know well in advance of having to make those choices, in order to find and select facilities that are compatible with our values. Which leads us to Opaque Dying Marketplace example three.

Opaque Dying Marketplace example, 2016: A Prevailing Absence of Basic Information

This third occurrence of the Opaque Dying Marketplace is not an instance, it's a backdrop. Only upon assessing it did the phrase Opaque Dying Marketplace finally occur to me, along with the analogy, "I'll show you mine if you'll show me yours."

Our advance directives, individually and collectively, are our personal and communal showing. We are showing medicine our most poignant, important desires about what we do and don't want to experience during life-threatening medical episodes and at the end of our lives. We present the documents upon demand. The trouble is, the moment of demand usually coincides with an existential, if not life-and-death, crisis; by then we're already in the thick of some situation (or landing, using the language of Windrum's Matrix), and our timeframe is no longer "advance"; rather, it's after the fact and right now!—a now in which we probably do not know the doctors' and institution's orientation to dying.

As is typical with this topic, there's much to unpack.

Today the idea of exerting personal control over our dying is becoming more mainstream; most of us are scared of experiencing protracted or mechanized deaths in institutional settings, and more medical professionals are tiring of (and saddened by) having to apply treatments that, when futile, actually equate to torture. In response, civilian political action has made medical aid in dying (MAID) legal in more jurisdictions. Voluntarily stopping eating and drinking (VSED) has emerged as an option of interest to dying people who may not qualify for MAID. (Pursuing VSED is best undertaken with some advance guidance; depending on one's condition it may or may not provide a pain-free, peaceful pathway. See Appendix C for several resources.) As a result, more people wonder what types of dying services local doctors, businesses, facilities, and institutions may offer. The Facebook group Slow Medicine, with over 4,000 civilian and professional members at this writing, hosts an increasing number of conversations posing this question in one form or another; other groups do too.

Although still a minority, a sizable percentage of civilians have heard and responded; we are taking the concept of advance planning to heart. Why can't civilians obtain a simple, honest, uniform answer to some basic questions about available end-of-life services where they live? Isn't asking and answering questions a core purpose of advance planning? We want to become more death-literate patients and proxies. What more basic place to begin than to ask of the doctors, businesses, facilities, and institutions around us: What type of end-of-life services do you offer? Please tell us in advance, so we don't have to wait to learn the answer until we risk infringement on peaceful dying because we've trekked too far into our dying territory. Do you offer a full spectrum of approaches to medically managed dying? Do you omit some? Do you offer aided dying where it's legal? Can I trust you not to remove life supports if we desire that they remain in place, to the extent allowed by law?

The latter two questions indicate interest in the most liberal and the most conservative end-of-life pathways. I summarize the range of approaches to end-of-life services and propose five broad categories, named to reveal the relationship to dying:

Welcoming | Accepting | Cautious | Resistant | Denying

Briefly described, a Welcoming approach would include transparent engagement with aided-dying statutes. An Accepting approach would champion palliative treatments, the early inclusion of patient-family values as part of medical decision-making, and full and early use of hospice. A Cautious approach would promote curative treatments to some length. A Resistant approach would resist death by engaging in successive ongoing treatment attempts, steering patient-families away from death acceptance. A Denying approach would virtually demand that the dying be kept on life supports for as long as could legally be sustained.

Any medical provider, individual or business, could indicate which of these five approaches they offer and which, if any, they do not offer (although they are not medically exclusive, I have to wonder how many institutions would provide all five dying services due to their divergence). The most relevant aspects could be summarized in bullet points below a simple five-column graphic. The many details governing end-of-life services would continue being communicated and negotiated during direct personal encounters. A simple chart would allow all of us to consider, essentially to shop, in advance. It would save everyone, civilian and professional alike, time and energy. Like would seek like; opposites would not engage unknowingly, only to discover amidst the tangle of dying that ethical chasms between patient-family and doctor/facility preclude a peaceful dying experience for the family and satisfying attendance by medical professionals.

Can you easily and quickly identify doctors and businesses with whom you might be interested in sharing an end-of-life journey (give your end-of-life business to), and those who you might want to avoid? Can you find this basic yet meaningful service range statement in brochures, on facility walls, on websites? Can you find it beside promises of "care" and pictures meant to convey promises of a peaceful experience?

Opaque Dying Marketplace example, 2017:
A Prominent Medical System's Chaplain Declines to Respond

Although I actively helped to pass Colorado's 2016 citizen initiative legalizing medical aid in dying, the Colorado End-of-Life Options Act, I didn't expect to participate as soon as I did after the law took effect in January 2017. That summer a 90-year-old friend asked me to serve as a witness to their application form for physician-aided dying. Subsequently I had a ringside seat to one patient-family's travails at they attempted to use the new state law.

This example of opacity in the dying marketplace is itself opaque, for I must describe its circumstances using stilted wording. A large regional medical system has published, in an easily found online format, that it would opt in to the Colorado End-of-Life Options Act which took effect January 1, 2017. Despite this, neither the facility, the clinic involved, nor the doctor involved want to publicize that they have made themselves available. To protect what access exists, I will describe events in more general terms than I would prefer, masking in strange wording details of gender, ailment, and facility and doctor identification. That I must do so within a discussion exemplifying the impact of the Opaque Dying Marketplace is an irony not lost on me. This is part of opacity's impact. The following two paragraphs contain the obfuscating wording and its twisted writing serves as an ironic example when we are not at liberty to transparently discuss end-of-life matters. I could shield identities by making up names, genders, pronouns, and medical conditions but I'd rather that we all experience the contortions forced upon us.

My friend and their adult child/surrogate had great difficulty finding doctors to engage with them. They were a patient of an organ specialist with a local office who is associated with a prominent medical system, itself located an hour's drive across a congested metropolitan area. A year prior, they had undergone invasive surgery intended to rejuvenate the patient; its effects quickly waned and left them more depleted than before the procedure. This nearly resulted in their landing in Progressed or Endstage Medically managed dying (in the language of Windrum's Matrix). The organ specialist and other local doctors declined to engage my friend about aided dying; doctors have that right under the law. They did not refer my friend to doctors who might. The system's organ specialty clinic initially also declined to facilitate engagement on the grounds that my friend was not a clinic patient (such status was required in order for an engaging physician to qualify as an attending physician under the terms of the Act).

Eventually, the surrogate convinced the clinic director that the parent's status as an organ failure patient of the local associate was sufficient for their intake into the system's organ specialty clinic. They were finally able to access a willing doctor. The time spent searching for willing doctors and then negotiating this status took well over a month. This was long enough to impact and almost imperil the patient's physical ability to meet all of the Act's requirements and might have thrown this patient-family into Failed dying (in the language of Windrum's Matrix). The delay, coupled with the need to arrange multiple trips across the metro region for the requisite evaluation meetings, added to this dying person's hardship.

Based on prior research during and after writing *Notes from the Waiting Room: Managing a Loved One's End-of-Life Hospitalization*, I learned and have subsequently advised that the medical chaplaincy is a particularly valuable resource for solving problems arising when we are involved with large medical institutions. Every chaplain whom I've met and queried reinforces this assertion enthusiastically.

So, curious, after my friend's death I contacted the chaplain at the system where my friend's quest for aided-dying assistance almost failed. For the first time, a chaplain whitewalled my query.

I may have asked the wrong question, for even with the knowledge that I've acquired, every engagement as a medical question-asker begins anew. I asked if the chaplain would have helped my friend connect with a willing doctor in the system had the friend approached the chaplain and asked. Via email, I received a vague reply extolling the general availability of the chaplaincy. It was a non-answer, so I wrote back, offering more of the story's details and requesting a response to the question I'd posed. I got no reply. After leaving voicemail I received a curt one-line reply that the system's chaplains do not refer patients to providers.

I should have asked if the chaplain would have helped to break a logjam between the seeking patient and the clinic denying their patient status and access to the service. But it's not incumbent upon us civilians to have the same knowledge as medical professionals; it ought to be incumbent upon medical professionals to evaluate the sort of detail-embellished query I'd finally made and to provide a meaningful answer to the conundrum.

To be fair, in any state with newly-enacted medical aid in dying laws, it takes time for access to normalize for many reasons: disinclination of even willing doctors to become overly sought for this purpose; administrative delays as medical systems decide whether to opt out or to opt in and, if the latter, to develop internal policies for engagement; a lack of public and professional education about these laws' clauses; absent clinical training in the art of assessing the optimum mix and dose of life-ending agents; and confusion by the public regarding the rights and responsibilities of all involved, which result in people waiting too long to apply. (See Appendix C for an extended discussion of these matters.)

Further research about this issue in my town yielded pleasant surprises: a softening of the Opaque Dying Marketplace. The chaplain at a different major medical system that's opted into Colorado's aided-dying law cheerfully and fully engaged with me. The chaplain at another system, which has opted out, advised me that they don't refer patients to specific providers, but we shared a ranging conversation. The provider/insurer Kaiser Permanente has opted in, and a director who is in charge of overseeing aided-dying requests from their subscribers spoke openly, albeit discretely, with me. And, during an unplanned conversation while shopping for a new primary physician as I approached Medicare age, a geriatric clinic's practice manager volunteered without prompting that everyone at the clinic supports aided dying and would work with patients who desire it. I am delighted to be able to close this contemporary example of the Opaque Dying Marketplace with an instance of voluntary transparency, which we deserve and will make all our lives easier. Such openness will humanize the end of life, and lead toward peace.

As a friend researched area hospices on behalf of a dying friend of his, he eventually located what is, at this writing, the only area hospice willing to facilitate medically aided dying on behalf of their own patients. As with my geriatrician's office, the hospice medical director volunteered their willingness before my friend could ask (although the doctor subsequently declined to be interviewed by a local reporter writing an article on the state of aided dying in our region on its first-year anniversary). No matter what one thinks of medically aided dying, I wonder, now that it's legal, if it's helping to stimulate a little less opacity, at least for medical professionals for whom protracted dying is not considered to be the necessary cost of extended living.

— —

The *Opacum Emporium Mortis* is insidious, harmful, cruel, and defeating. It's time for medicine to "show us theirs." To state their preferences in the same manner and timeframe in which they urge us to state ours. To disclose, when we ask, policies affecting our dying experiences—especially while we're healthy enough to incorporate their answers into our advance planning. To communicate their range of end-of-life service offerings, so that we may understand the basic contours in advance and judge if we should enter into a dying relationship with a given organization, facility, or doctor, or look elsewhere. Medicine's reticence to disclose its members' orientations around dying erects a barrier to society becoming death-literate, accepting of death, wiser about approaching and living our final days. Dying in peace requires, in part, a transparent dying marketplace as we plan for and make our way home.

Unless and until medicine broadly shows us theirs, we have no solution to the obstacle thrown up by the Opaque Dying Marketplace other than to name it, know it's all around us, and challenge it when it looms before us. We must exert pressure to influence medicine to show us theirs—to state and explain their orientation toward end-of-life treatment delivery and to reveal and explain their policies. Each of us must ask doctors and administrators to do so at every relevant medical encounter, in any medical environment, again and again—before we or our loved ones are actually dying.

To Die in Peace: Our Rights of Passage Recap

Awareness of these practical, everyday obstacles to peaceful dying is the first step to overcoming them. Let's put them together as an all-inclusive question. If I:

- [Am subject to conflicted family relations, restrictive beliefs, or financial duress, and]

- Lack the language to distinguish among the array of dying situations,

- Cannot assess when enough medically heroic engagement is enough,

- Feel complacent because I have advance directives, and then…

- Become at risk of experiencing medical snafus: misadventure and/or medical error,

- Get snagged by life-support overrides, and

- Fail to advocate effectively,

- In an opaque dying marketplace,

- Where might I land?

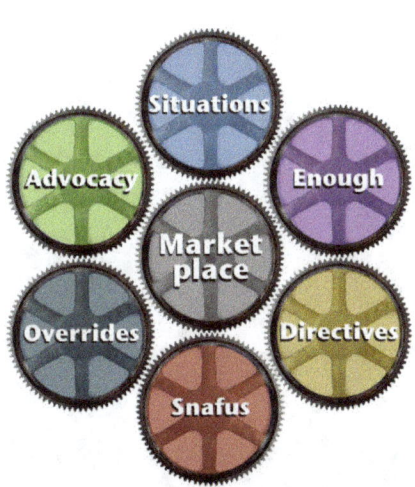

It's up to each of us to answer these questions for ourselves. As of this writing, the majority of Americans have not executed advance directives and at least half of us remain at high risk of experiencing peace-less, overmedicalized demises. Hospice enrollments are increasing, albeit much later in the dying process than is maximally beneficial and legally available. Awareness of palliative medicine as a beneficial adjunct to, and even replacement for, late-life Hail Mary efforts to sustain unsustainable lives is increasing. Death doulas and green burial options indicate a slowly percolating public movement toward death literacy. The trend line appears to be moving in what many end-of-life reform advocates consider the right direction. Yet patient-family experiences of hospice, both for-profit and non-profit, are increasingly subject to the inhumane aspects of corporatization; the U.S. implementation of electronic health record systems and the growing corporatization of medical institutions are decimating doctors' ability to attend to the patients in front of them; U.S. insurers find ever more devious ways to shift medical costs onto policyholders; and little if any systemic support, let alone payment, for caregivers exists. We'd be foolish to presume peaceful dying as a norm, or to abandon our proactive, protective vigilance if peaceful dying is our goal.

Our 21st Century End-of-life Milieu

Modern obstacles to peaceful dying exist within a larger end-of-life milieu. The top gear set depicts the end-of-life totality in simpler times—most of human history; these elemental aspects remain our fundamental experience. The bottom gear set represents conventional modern guidance for people wanting to minimize their exposure to the downside risks of late life medical overtreatment. The middle gear contains aspects of 21st century dying that most of us encounter briefly or at length, smoothly or with difficulty. These interrelated obstacles to peaceful dying are an inescapable part of engagement with modern medicine; spinning the bottom gear set and experiencing the top gear set inevitably engages the middle realm and its internal gears—personal and systemic obstacles to peaceful dying.

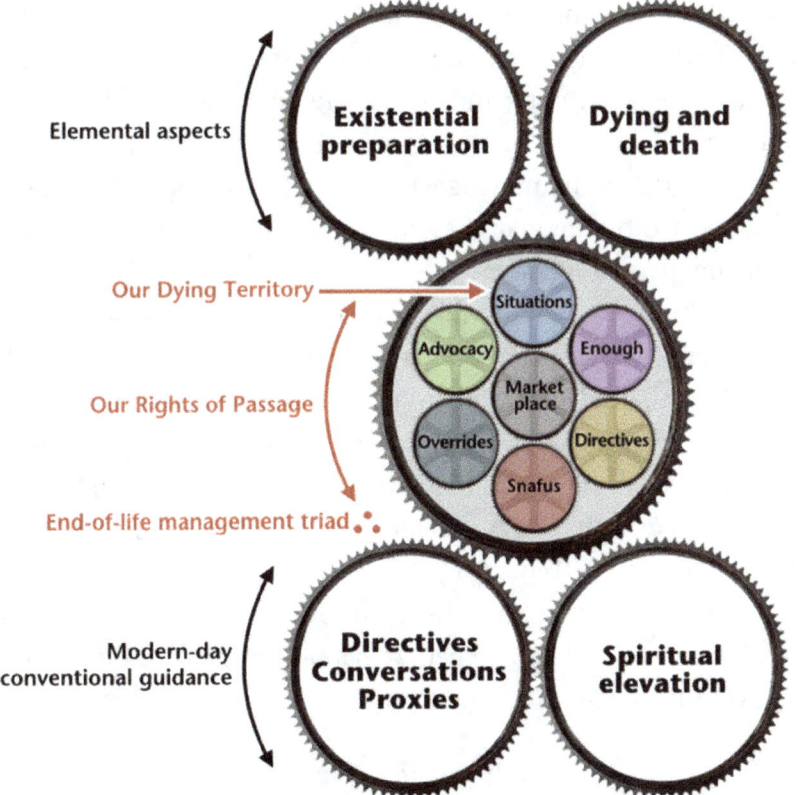

Chapter 11

Deus Ex Machina?

I hope, sincerely, that you are now metaphorically enjoying some lemonade, sweetened just enough by knowing that you've acquired some useful knowledge. I understand if you might feel a bit dubious at the suggestion that this unflinching look at how our society shapes dying has an enjoyable aspect. Please know that all my work since 2004 does not cause me to feel sanguine or masterful. I am not looking forward, at all, to the next time I must engage medically about these matters. My own fear of failure is grounded in knowing that I tend not to be smart in real time, under duress; that I tend toward a short fuse and the absence of anything approaching equanimity; and my deep resentment that any of us—let alone all of us—are subject to everything this book addresses. Yet I take comfort in knowing what I have come to know, and feeling supported by the many resources available now that were not during my parents' demises.

I won't do what I'm asking medicine to stop doing—paint an unreasonably rosy picture when a prognosis is known to be mixed, pretending that all is OK when all is not OK. I think that medicine's behavior and our civilian cohort's behavior around death and dying will remain variable, better in some instances and worse in others. We won't know which describes ours until we are in the thick of events. Few of us, if any, will benefit from a deus ex machina, a miracle ending where irreconcilable aspects go conveniently unaddressed and somehow happily resolved, a crazy (and lazy) theatrical and cinematic technique known as the "god from the machine"—a contrived solution to an apparently insoluble difficulty (Merriam-Webster).

Having read *The Promised Landing*, you are in a better position than you were before. You are aware of obstacles that you were formerly unaware of, or perhaps sensed but couldn't articulate. This book alone has not provided you with all the details and skills to advocate medically, but you now have a vital baseline: sensitized foresight. Your antennae are up, sensitive to what you perceive when you look at our dying territory. You might notice a word, an inflection, a reticence to answer, an implication in something said or unsaid by loved ones as well as medical professionals, an unasked question begging to be answered. Some absence where there should be some presence. Some act about to occur that you know ought not to occur. Inadequate attention when competent attention is required. Something will catch your attention, you'll stop and really notice. You'll ask yourself, "Is there a looming problem ahead, an obstacle in our glide path to peaceful dying? Is this the moment, right now, that I must begin acting to mitigate that obstacle so as to maintain our glide path, to make our landing?" From here on, your sensitivity is your guide.

And so, at age 65, I advance in a mixed state, with a tenuous hope for peace as our society begins a broad-based effort to understand what we've done to dying and death, and what this condition has done to us. I hope that *The Promised Landing* helps you and your loved ones achieve what my elder loved ones and I failed to achieve. I hope it helps us all, in poet Rainer Maria Rilke's words, to "be ahead of all parting"* when our time comes to part with our loved ones and our lives on planet Earth.

---

* The Sonnets To Orpheus, Part 2, Sonnet XIII, Stephen Mitchell translation

"I might experience peaceful dying."

"I might experience peace-less dying."

"I might experience peaceful dying."

And So

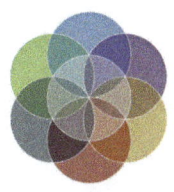

Appendix A

The Rusted Gate

The rusted gate, a metaphor I used in this book's opening (on page 8), has its genesis in a poem I wrote in response to a type and intensity of introspection peculiar, I believe, to men. Men's Work and men's groups emerged in the 1990s. In my community small, regular gatherings focused on eliciting deep, authentic relationship. This poem was written after a barrage of unexpectedly severe criticism from a man to whom I had opened my own rusted emotional gate. The poem contains an interesting reference to the end of life, an unusual inclusion at age 41, 11 years before I experienced death in my immediate family. Although not its original focus, *Sweating Oil* conveys the uncomfortable aspects of becoming death-literate and the brave, humane work death literacy requires.

Sweating Oil

I held open the rusted gate
he came inside, Sherlock Holmes, all looking glass,
and observed what anyone could observe
with the naked eye
Attributes, disliked but not hidden,
in dusty corners thus defiled:
magnified into horrific proportions under a scrutiny
only the introspective endure
Although a puff would have sufficed
his blizzard exposed what was always exposed
to the rusted hail of our bitterness

Yes, this gate needs oiling
I sweat oil in my dreams
Dreams of stones dislodged; gates—
a mobius strip of gates, each one opening
this way and that way; a double-helix mobius of gates—
To blend science and metaphor in this new age,
which so reminds me of the old,
when, small, I stooped,
powerless against the hail's precedent

Man, take these stones, the ones I dreamt I moved
the sack you carry will be the same sack you always carry
We are given our gravestones at birth
and a lifetime in which to set them

Should these gates wave wildly at your passing, as if arms,
they are
If the airs thus stirred touch clumsily, childlike,
they are
When winds intone inexhaustible sorrow,
they are

Men's Work 1993, and under the influence of Rilke, revised

Appendix B

Never Say Die Rap

Coincident with preparing my 2013 TEDxFoCo talk, another wholly unexpected end-of-life work emerged. At first it was too weird. I've grown to love it.

Poetry and music simultaneously condense and enlarge what they give voice to. The Never Say Die Rap says much about end-of-life matters in a wonderfully compact form. Setting it to music was a thrill for me, a drummer who played a ragtag jimmy-rigged "kit" throughout my elementary school years and a 13-drum professional drum set for my last public ensemble performance during the summer of 1985 at Denver City Park's Pavilion. For the Rap, I found the right sound loop (DJ Buzzword's Danger Zone), changed its tempo without changing its pitch, added spare melodic orchestration using Apple's GarageBand software, overdubbed the final multipart chorus, and added a syncopated percussion line performed live with red sparkle drumsticks. The whole enterprise was and remains a hoot. Yet the Rap is a serious tool that communicates a distilled essence of our systemically absurd end-of-life conundrum. Rap about that...

The performance is contained within my TEDxFoCo video, from 7:50–10:10, viewable at AxiomAction.com/speaking. Or at YouTube.com search for "Windrum TEDxFoCo."

Never Say Die Rap

Want to die at peace got to die in peace
All of one piece say "pretty please"
Want to go in grace with a neutral face
We're done this race—NO got to stay in place
Beyond ready to depart
Jump jack your bones and shock your heart
When you're pickin pickin at the air
No bro' ma'am you ain't goin nowhere

Never Say Die Rap

There's an app for that
Never Say Die Rap

Independent thinker, no one's rube
Shove in 1 2 3 4 5 tubes
With CDiff MRSA gurgle gurgle
And all I wanna do is cuddle and snuggle
There's no app for that
Never Say Die Rap

And: in the annals of stupidity
Death panels twist our talkin free
Can't touch the sky, see or be seen
Ain't livin ain't dyin don't mean to be mean
When death comes knockin my clock tic tockin
Hey everybody: deus ex machina?
Rap about that...
Never Say Die Rap

Now it ain't just medicine in our way
If you don't talk, you don't get no say
Call 9-1-1 when it's time to pass
Blockin our own path, pain in our own ass
Take a number for that!
Never Say Die Rap

My friend Steve Price RN sings dyin is dyin
His songs are cool, Steve ain't lyin
Chart your glide path while there's time
To die in peace with minimal cryin
Study up, make some sense
Of 21st century impediments
Time to grow up before we get old
There's more to dying than we've been told
Wishing won't help us turn the page
So 17 new terms to engage
I have a Matrix for that...
Never Say Die Rap

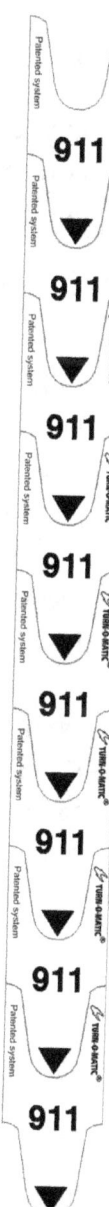

Appendix C

On Advocating

Books from many authors, both civilian and medical, offer guidance for advocating through late life and through medical emergencies. *The Promised Landing* focuses not on learning how to advocate, but on learning what we need to advocate about. Because effective advocacy is so important, this Appendix offers a short course in the aspects of medical advocacy that I deem most useful given this book's content.

Independent Thinker, No One's Rube:
Ending at the Beginning

Because everything starts with the basics, it's useful to revisit them. This end-of-life lexicon's taproot is a redefinition of what medicine provides. It is not "care," and the fact that it is not is why I attempt to avoid using the term "healthcare." Everything in *The Promised Landing* emanates from the following statement expressing, from the civilian perspective, what medicine does provide. Understanding this is crucial to effective advocacy because it orients us toward stepping into our role as surrogates before we're immersed in it during some crisis.

> Medicine does not provide care;
> medicine provides bodily repair services
> under the direction of independent physician-scientists
> and nurse-monitoring on some schedule.

Here's how this understanding came about. In early 2004, my mother Ruth's sudden respiratory collapse became the onset of her demise. After nearly a week in a compassionless intensive care setting, my father, my sister (a neonatal intensive care nurse), and I had become uneasy. We didn't understand the rationale for much of what was happening, and couldn't understand why obvious aspects of Ruth's care lapsed. I found myself musing about care, for we did not feel cared for in the slightest. Nor did we feel that Mom was receiving careful treatment due to the daily errors we observed and tried to mitigate. I strove to understand what exactly we were receiving, if not health-*care*. My thoughts ran this way because I knew that we were not supporting my mother as best as we ought to or could. What had we been waiting for all week long? What had we been receiving? We had been waiting for care, to be cared for. We were receiving something different, absent anything like care as we understood the term. Initially, my thinking included only in-hospital doctoring. After Dad's hospitalized demise and a family member's midlife hospitalization, I included nursing. I've come to apply the definition of what medicine provides to medicine as a social edifice. At this writing (2018), I must also acknowledge that some physicians may no longer function independently; more doctors are becoming employees of hospital systems, beholden to imperatives of corporately-controlled medicine.

With this understanding we can orient ourselves to perform the work that medicine, through its unified statements, tells us to do: advocate for ourselves or as proxies for our loved ones. It's a serious job performed in difficult circumstances, in situations we wish we weren't in, by people who are inexpert, for longer periods of time than we want to endure. We can't afford to lose any time during serious medical circumstances; the sooner we understand our role and task, the better for all involved.

Nothing about this redefinition disrespects medical professionals or precludes individuals from working care-fully or manifesting care as sons and daughters, brothers and sisters, lovers and friends know and understand care. Any one of us, anytime, anywhere, doing anything can compassionately offer ourselves through our work with what I call in *Notes from the Waiting Room* "mom and apple pie care."

It is possible that a hospitalized death in a kindly, supportive facility with ready resources has the potential to be more peaceful than a home death lacking a robust support network and a fully responsive hospice agency. For most of us, I think it safe to say that the best way to manage a terminal hospitalization is not to have one. The conundrum is that it is also possible that the end-of-life peace we seek may end up being equal to the peace lost seeking it. Such are the complexities and unknowns in our fragmented, convoluted health "care" system.

Can't Touch the Sky:
Advance Directives

This section is not a discussion detailing advance directives, the need for them, their utility (or not), or the challenges and considerations around formulating them. Here I simply list and briefly describe a number of directives that U.S. residents may want to consider. As the list shows, the options go beyond the basics (Living Will, surrogate assignment).

I am not a lawyer; what follows is not legal advice. That said, my viewpoint is that we must plug every hole we can imagine opening in the safety net these documents are meant to weave, no matter how loose that weave may be.

You may change or override your own directives by voice or in writing anytime. As long as you are conscious and mentally competent, what you say goes, each time, every time, in real time. Conversely, nobody else should be able to override your directives anytime. The sole exception is medical professionals under distinct circumstances where the law and medicine claim to have a higher right than you (a debatable concept but one that is, in fact, in effect to differing degrees in different situations).

If we are to be smart, we will consider directives mandatory for all adults of legal age. This is not to say they will be available, found, read, understood, put into effect, and protect us according to what we set forth in them. But only those who know that they want every lifesaving medical intervention applied without fail would live without them. Personally, I would have every document witnessed and notarized every time (excepting doctors' orders) to minimize the chances that someone, somewhere, sometime, somehow, would attempt to challenge or discredit one of the directives.

Medical Durable Power of Attorney The MDPOA is used to designate a health care surrogate, a person or persons you trust to represent you and direct your medical treatment should you become incapable of doing so yourself. At its broadest, unless you specify limits, your surrogate will have full legal powers over medical matters pertaining to you: interacting with providers; rejecting, accepting, and directing all medical treatments; accessing all your medical records (both historical and current); and making life-and-death decisions. "Durable" means that these powers remain in force after your death (this is pertinent for accessing medical records).

HIPAA Authorization and Release HIPAA, the Health Insurance Portability and Accountability Act, is the U.S. federal government's framework meant to protect our medical privacy. Over time, it seems to have been turned against us, creating roadblocks for managing our own treatment with the assistance of our spouses and surrogates. An increasing quagmire, we're confronted with provider unwillingness to give us and our surrogates access to our own medical information unless we jump through their specific hoops. Although HIPAA matters can be addressed within a surrogate directive, some lawyers suggest having a separate HIPAA authorization/release document. While most doctors' offices, in my experience, prefer and even demand that we fill out their one-off HIPAA authorization/release forms (useful only for each specific practice or clinic), the day may come when a patient who hasn't done that becomes incapable of doing it. I like having my lawyer-drafted universal HIPAA authorization/release form in my suite of directives should my surrogates ever need to, literally, brandish it. No matter what practice managers may say, a lawyer-drafted, correctly executed HIPAA authorization/release directive is legally binding and executable.

A surrogate assignment without a corresponding HIPAA designation is, in my opinion, a very risky scenario; I can imagine certain circumstances under which a legal surrogate could be denied access to their principal's medical record. These directives are your protection and are legal business; cross all the Ts and dot all the Is. Get HIPAA handled or run a risk of crippling your surrogate's ability to advocate on your behalf.

Living Will   A Living Will is the classic end-of-life directive. It can be formal or informal. It may be pre-structured (Five Wishes is particularly well known) or one's own narrative in the form of a letter. It ought to be, in my opinion, a brief-as-possible, values-based document expressing what constitutes a life worth continuing and where one draws the line to stop medical treatments. Providers may not prefer such a document because it's hard to quickly find specific directives to allow or disallow various treatments. I find creating a values-based Living Will to be exceedingly challenging and recommend looking for seminars offered by reputable end-of-life counselors to help facilitate one's exploration and subsequent expression within a Living Will. Other names for similar directives include Values Directive and Letter to My Doctor.

Financial Durable Power of Attorney   The FDPOA is not usually listed as part of end-of-life advance planning directives. Clearly, health and medical matters present a risk of intersecting with financial matters. If a surrogate were to need money to pay for medical services or products, they ought to be able to get it. This directive ought to accompany one's traditional (property) will or trust documents anyway.

Resuscitation Order   Currently, there are two levels of resuscitation directives. The classic original is the Do Not Resuscitate Order, or DNR. Throughout the United States, DNRs are being superseded by POLST, COLST, MOST, and other flavors of "OLST" forms. The Physician Orders for Life-Sustaining Treatment, Clinical Orders for Life-Sustaining Treatment, or Medical Orders for Scope of Treatment forms list a range of resuscitation and life-sustaining treatments in a checkbox format inside visually boxed sections. When filled in, the idea is that one's range of allowables and disallowables is quickly and easily understandable without having to read through paragraphs and pages as with a Living Will. Civilians cannot make anti-resuscitation orders on our own behalf; only doctors can (a restriction on personal liberty which distinctly annoys me). And DNRs and "OLST" forms are meant for people whose health is highly compromised or are severely ill, terminally ill, or dying. The doctor's signature on any of these forms makes them medical orders that emergency responders and other medical providers are legally and duty-bound to honor, providing that the forms are completed in good order and brought to their attention.

Allow Natural Dying Order The AND directive is another flavor of resuscitation directive. It focuses a little more on the positive ("allow"). It's a kinder, gentler way of expressing anti-resusciation choices. As with DNRs and POLSTs, a doctor's signature is required.

Dementia Directive A dementia directive sets forth, while one is mentally competent, limits on allowable treatments in the event of future dementia when one would not be able to express such thoughts. The directive could be a simple standalone document with the same choices/checkboxes listed three times, once each for mild, moderate, and severe dementia. Or, we might specifically address dementia in a separate section within a living will or values directive.

Do Not Transport Directive If you or a loved one lives in a residential facility, especially one that is corporately owned, and do not want to be taken to an emergency room or a hospital in the event of a severe medical downturn, fill out this form and file it with the facility and with your surrogate(s).

Sectarian Hospitals Directive If you disagree with limits that the Catholic Church places on personal choice regarding late-life medical treatments and do not want yourself, your family, and your doctors to be subject to them, fill out this form, add it to your directives suite, and file it with your surrogates. First responders typically take people to the nearest facility capable of handling the medical condition/s afflicting the person they're transporting. Should that end up being a Catholic facility or one governed by a Catholic organization (which may not be immediately evident, you'll have to ask...), you might want to be transferred to a facility that is not affiliated with the Church. This directive gives your surrogates the explicit right to attempt to make that transfer.

Assisted-living Rider If you are concerned about the potential for degraded living or treatment conditions in an assisted-living facility, consider executing a rider setting forth your requirements and parameters and adding it to your residency agreement documents at signing. I do not know if these businesses would accept and agree to your terms or not, but the need for such a rider has been raised among patient activists. I find it reasonable, and so include the option here.

Feeding Directive Engaging in the type of reflection that medicine urges regarding the formulation of advance directives, some peoples' attention has turned to feeding issues. For some, arriving at the point of refusal of food is a benchmark indicating that life quality has declined to a point that death is preferable to extended living. A feeding directive might require caregivers to honor various patient expressions of food refusal, disallowing repetitive or aggressive attempts at feeding. I recommend a long conversation with some number of nurses plus civilians with prior experience in order to assess the range of feeding approaches and interventions that ought to be addressed by a feeding directive.

Hospital Visitation Directive If you feel the need to control who may participate in the social goings-ons during hospitalizations, this is the directive to use. Specify people you explicitly want to allow into the circle around you and/or to disallow from being present, mingling, voicing opinions, disrupting, and otherwise attempting to influence events.

Call 911 When It's Time to Pass?
Understanding 911 and Obtaining Assistance

The provision of emergency assistance is governed by an institutional approach to emergency responsiveness: maintain biological life ("save lives") in all cases, do it quickly, and ask questions after the fact. 911 Emergency Response is a blunt instrument. Those employed as its agents are not charged with making fine distinctions. They may, or may not, be up-to-date; they may be unaware that POLST and MOST regulations have taken legal effect in their jurisdictions and may not know that these forms exist. Responders ought to be trained to ask for directives and to know the several common places to quickly look for them (wallet/purse; stuck to the refrigerator, or on an inside wall beside the front door). Know, however, that in life-and-death situations, seconds count, decisions are made rapidly, and second-guessing takes a backseat to lifesaving no matter the downstream consequences. Calling 911 is not like asking a neighbor for help around the house; it is literally a call to and for a multi-alarm response. Even if it's not a life-and-death emergency, the responders will come with sirens blaring and adrenaline flowing.

The cliché is true: a strong bias exists for transport to hospital emergency rooms and from there into hospital wards. This pathway is appropriate in some instances and may be extraordinarily inappropriate in others. The vignette I presented as representative of Emergency Room dying in chapter 8 is based on a true story of a dying man's wife having called 911 in the wee hours because she had no one else to call; all she wanted was assistance getting her husband, who had fallen returning to bed from the bathroom, back into bed. The old guy was literally several days from death. Instead, alarmed at his obvious condition and ignoring the wife's attempt to explain their circumstances and intentions, responders carted him off to the ER. He was admitted to the hospital, and both he and his wife suffered massive extrinsic shock and promise pain as he succumbed to in-hospital Endstate dying instead of the independent, at-home death they'd assiduously planned for and worked toward. They would have done better to bundle him up, have him finish the night on the floor, and find non-emergency help in the morning.

On the basis of that story, I ask the following questions quite literally: Is it OK to die with our butts on the floor? Is it dignified, is it reasonable, is it acceptable, to die on the floor between the bed and the wall? Is this better or worse than experiencing institutionalized end days that the man and wife in our vignette experienced? What is required of us in order to increase our likelihood of dying in, and at, peace?

And why did they experience being carted off? Because we have a one-size brute force red-alert response system. We do not have a tiered, less-than-emergency, assistive response resource. It's possible that some localities may be attempting to create a nuanced assistive resource. Call your county government (probably their senior services department) and inquire.

Lastly, popular TV shows have drastically misinformed us by portraying "code blue" resuscitations as much less brutal and far more effective than they are in real life. Especially for elders, rates of success are very slim (less than 5% to 15%). Even then, "success" is defined as the person not having died. In most cases, injury and substantial post-resuscitation decline in ability and quality of life are the norm. In other words, elders generally come out the backside of a "successful" resuscitation in worse, if not far worse, condition than before resuscitation was applied: literally, lesser men and women than before.

If You Don't Talk You Don't Get No Say: Medical Approaches to Seek

For those who would like to find medical professionals aligned with values like tapering medical treatments when age and condition raise the risks of medical misadventure, the following initiatives and specialties will be of interest. There are others; in the absence of national reform, civilians, local or regional medical systems, and communities are left to their own devices to promote and formulate change.

The following approaches to late-life medical matters are ones that I know about and which resonate for me. Palliative and geriatric doctors and practices may not be as readily suggested as surgical specialists, or as available, especially when a serious illness presents. Hospice is widely known, yet misunderstood and under-utilized despite increasing enrollment. And yet, its service capacity is spread thin. Slow Medicine, Choosing Wisely, and Right Care are new initiatives gaining traction in the medical space and among in-the-know civilians. To connect with medical professionals practicing or oriented toward these methods, we have to ask for them. "If you don't talk you don't get no say," so ask to be connected with doctors of the following persuasions. While all medical professionals should know about geriatrics, palliation, and hospice, expect few to know about Slow Medicine, Choosing Wisely, and Right Care. Doctors who know about or are involved in these initiatives may be the ones you're looking to partner with.

Geriatric Medicine Geriatric medicine is a medical subspecialty focusing on the treatment and care of people 60 to 65 years of age and older. Geriatricians specialize in conditions of aging and how those conditions interact, including medications. Geriatric doctors function as primary care providers, including coordinating the engagement of other medical specialists. With a greater acceptance of the aged and their quirks, and a softer outlook toward providing medical treatments, geriatric medicine is in alignment with those wanting to aim for gentler end-of-life landings.

Palliative Care Palliative care is a medical subspecialty that reformers wish could be established as medicine's foundation, with primary care and other specialties arrayed underneath a palliative umbrella. As it is, palliative care, if known at all, is too-often misconstrued with giving up on life, supposedly where medical castoffs go when technological intervention options run out (which could take a while, and the delay would shortchange people for whom palliative care can provide substantial and supportive treatments). Palliative care focuses on symptom management and the relief of suffering. It's associated with the end-of-life but has applications long before active dying. Surgical procedures intended to cure might be chosen for their palliative effect even well into a demise. Don't expect to be offered a palliative consultation; ask for one as early as a demise begins to evidence itself. You might consider asking for a palliative consult even as soon as receiving a diagnosis of a serious, life-limiting illness. Don't be deterred should people raise their eyebrows and exclaim that you're not dying yet; palliative care is quite misunderstood. It is, literally, good medicine, focused on supporting the most and best living possible during one's waning lifespan. Remember—"Want to die at peace, got to die in peace."

Hospice Hospice serves people who have been diagnosed as terminally ill (technically, expected by a doctor of having no more than six months to live) as well as their family members. The diagnosis is all that's needed to make application for hospice services, and one could have half a year or more of peaceful living with hospice assistance, assuming early enrollment. U.S. federal rules preclude pursuing curative medicine when on hospice, but palliative treatments (including surgeries) performed primarily to relieve discomfort are allowable even if they're the same surgeries used to attempt cures. Those waiting to enroll in hospice until the end of a long technological demise (Endstate, Suspended, and Repetitive dying in terms of Windrum's Matrix) will severely underutilize hospice's ability to help us die in peace. That said, variations in staffing, service offerings, and profit orientation negatively impact many hospices' ability to adequately serve the dying, so shop carefully; don't be swayed solely by lovely images meant to convey a sense of peace. Although the boundaries may blur during very late life, hospice is not a substitute for other assistance with daily living and everyday caregiving. Do not expect round-the-clock services; do expect to provide your own support for dying family and friends. And do expect to have to advocate throughout a demise in the same manner required during hospitalizations.

Given how important hospice is, an article contemporary to my writing this section, titled "Hospice in Crisis," may be useful. It discusses hospice's history and its possible futures, some of them being introduced at this writing. It's worth a read: http://politico.com/agenda/story/2017/09/27/how-hospice-works-000526

Slow Medicine   Slow Medicine is a movement that started in Italy following that country's Slow Food movement for savoring nutritious ingredients and slow-paced meals, and the Slow Cities designation for cities banning automobiles from central plazas. The late geriatrician, Dennis McCullough (who authored *My Mother, Your Mother: Embracing Slow Medicine*) was among the first U.S. proponents. The physician-author Victoria Sweet has authored a memoir, *Slow Medicine: The Way to Healing*, recounting her embrace of it. As previously mentioned, Facebook's Slow Medicine group founded by author Katy Butler is a particularly vibrant online community of knowledgeable, solution-seeking civilians, doctors and nurses, end-of-life ethicists, death doulas, and others, where discussion of many Slow Medicine and end-of-life matters flows informatively, compassionately, and freely.

In *My Mother, Your Mother*, Dennis McCullough suggests that a "circle of concern" made up of health professionals, the patient-family, close friends, and select others join in supporting each aging individual. The Slow Medicine orientation tends to "moderate the urgent pressures of decision-making that are often pushed prematurely on elders by society, the medical professional, worried friends, and family." Doctors and nurses practicing Slow Medicine will pay "deep attention" to patients as people with histories. Because Slow Medicine is not inherently anti-medical intervention, it takes into account the full range of factors making up one's condition. A related aspect is to remain free of institutionalization, "aging in place" in our homes. Resources for doing so may be available from or tracked by U.S. county governments.

Not all doctors will be aware of Slow Medicine, but those who are conversant with its precepts may be attempting to work them into their medical practices. Slow Medicine does not repudiate traditional Western medicine ("fast medicine"), it incorporates and balances its strengths while moderating its weaknesses.

Choosing Wisely Choosing Wisely is a campaign of the American Board of Internal Medicine. According to their website, "The effort has garnered the participation of over 70 medical specialty societies who have published more than 400 recommendations of overused tests and treatments that clinicians and patients should discuss. The campaign and society recommendations have been included in nearly 300 journal articles and more than 10,000 media articles since the program launched in 2012." *Consumer Reports*, in association with the campaign, has published a wide range of resources for civilians. Thus, there would seem to be some traction and bandwidth to this initiative.

Right Care Dr. Bernard Lown developed the original cardiac defibrillator. His work led to the formation of coronary care units. A longtime peace activist, Lown and colleagues in 2012 founded the Lown Institute, which addresses the interrelated problems of medical under-treatment, over-treatment, and mis-treatment. Right Care, the Institute's initiative to correct these problems, includes public outreach and clinical programs. As with Slow Medicine, not all doctors will know about Right Care, but those who do may be working to apply its principles to their medical practices.

From Lown Institute vice-president Shannon Brownlee's book, *Overtreated: Why Too Much Medicine is Making Us Sicker and Poorer*, Right Care principles may be expressed as a set of core questions we're encouraged to ask when medical treatments are proposed:
- What are my options?
- How exactly might the treatment help?
- What adverse ("side") effects can we expect, and what bad outcomes might happen?
- How good is the evidence that I might benefit from the treatment?
- If it's a test: what do we expect to learn from it, and how might it change my treatment?

— —

Related to these three initiatives, it's useful to carefully consider the advisability and utility of tests and procedures; at advanced age they may not be harmless. Some valid questions to ask include:
- Would you recommend this for your spouse, sibling, mother, or father?
- What happens if I don't undergo this test/procedure?
- What is the recommended treatment if this test results in bad news?
- Ask yourself if you would engage in the recommended treatment after a bad result. If not, should you undergo the test?

There is no one-size-fits-all in medicine, although in the United States federal payment is increasingly tied to benchmarks associated with what's known as evidence-based medicine. Some benchmarks are useful for swaths of a population, but the aging and aged, the "young old" and the very old, may fall outside those bounds based on common sense assessments of the entirety of their condition and lifespan. Palliative and geriatric medicine, hospice, Slow Medicine, Choosing Wisely, and Right Care are key approaches to seek. These approaches are especially important at the end of life, for dying in peace really means living our waning days as well and peacefully as we are able with the assistance of compassionately offered and sensibly applied medical treatments—no less and no more.

No Bro Ma'am You Ain't Goin' Nowhere:
On the Availability of Medical Aid in Dying

I support medical aid in dying despite its challenges and the shortcomings associated with its implementation. Yet it should be abundantly clear that To Die in Peace: Our Rights of Passage is not about aided dying. Obstacles to peaceful dying will persist no matter where aided dying becomes legal. Remember: dying in peace pertains to the months, weeks, and days of our demise, during which we likely will seek and need to manage medical treatments so as to obtain their benefits yet keep from getting dragged into dying situations we know we wish to avoid. Medical aid in dying (MAID), also known as physician-aided dying, is about choosing and controlling, insofar as possible, the moment we die—personally directing our dying to maximize our chance of dying in peace.

In our dying territory, represented by Windrum's Matrix of Dying Terms, MAID is successfully utilized when the patient-family experiences either Released or Postponed dying. Those who wait too long and can no longer meet the laws' requirements experience Failed dying—essentially a placeholder for Endstate, Suspended, Repetitive, or possibly Vegetative dying. For those who value and aim for aided dying, its availability matters, a lot.

I have long seen the emergence of aided dying as a logical civilian response to generations of overly hard dying afflicting millions of dying people and multiple millions more of their surviving loved ones. Think about these numbers—peace-less dying has become an epidemic. Civilians cannot change medicine; medical professionals can barely make a dent in medical culture and practice even when they're inclined to. Enacting medical aid in dying is one small change that citizens are successfully making in the end-of-life realm.

In Colorado, USA, where I live, I helped pass the Colorado End-of-Life Options Act by gathering signatures to place it on the ballot and by writing articles and editorials arguing for its passage. The law took effect late in 2016. As previously noted, six months after its passage, I was asked to serve as a witness on an elderly friend's request form used to initiate the process, and thus unexpectedly took a ringside seat to their family's travails in attempting to locate participating doctors at more-or-less the last minute. The same struggle to find willing doctors recurred three months later for a friend helping a friend navigate this new territory. So I have a fresh set of insights regarding challenges associated with implementing and accessing such a paradigm-shifting law.

Let's examine important aspects for those wanting to access medical-aid-in-dying services under newly-established laws. Since these laws involve both civilians and medical professionals, let's look at aspects that pertain to each group. What follows is informed by my exposure in general and by the statute where I live; details and aspects may differ in different jurisdictions.

Civilian Problems Accessing Medical Aid in Dying

The civilian sector appears to have several misapprehensions about aided dying. The first has to do with access to it. Essentially, people seem to think that gaining access to aided dying will be quick, as casual as purchasing some personal item. And that death after ingestion will be very fast (it may, or it may not...). And that some system for providing the service and products it requires will have been established when the law takes effect. And that medical systems and doctors support or even know about it.

If ever a law needed reading, your jurisdiction's aided-dying law is it. Google it, download it. If your computer skills allow, convert the hard-to-read all-capitalized legal document to sentence-caps (normal everyday capitalization). The Colorado End-of-Life Options Act runs 11 pages. It's an easy read. This webpage links to the legislative texts of existing laws: TheIrisProject.net/resources-on-physician-assisted-death.html

Aided dying is not a turnkey system. It is not immediately, universally, easily, or readily available. It's hard to access because we must find and become patients of doctors who are willing to engage. Doctors' engagement is *not* mandatory. Those who do so may not publicize their availability or want it publicized. This also applies to health systems with which doctors associate.

In general, to qualify one must be a resident of the jurisdiction. While no end-of-life medical "tourism" is allowed, gaining residency can be quick. If you live outside of the jurisdiction you'll need to research how to become a resident (don't expect MAID laws to detail how) and prove it when requesting MAID. One must be dying and diagnosed as such. Currently in all U.S. jurisdictions, you must be diagnosed by two physicians as terminal, with six months or less left to live. You must be mentally competent from start to finish (advanced dementia sufferers likely need not apply).

Practically speaking, one must be physically able to travel to and from the necessary appointments. One must be able to afford the cost of the prescribed drugs—do not be surprised if their cost magically multiplies in jurisdictions where MAID is being contemplated or has become law. One must be able to ingest the lethal prescription by oneself (others may help to prepare it). One should have at-home assistance (do not expect that hospitals will allow MAID to take place in their facilities). One may need to keep secrets to prevent unwanted interference from residents and management of corporate-owned shared living facilities, even if those entities have not banned MAID on their premises. Expect most hospices to decline participation or to take a very limited role in your personally-controlled death.

Finding willing health systems and doctors will probably take a lot of time, especially right after a law takes effect and possibly as an ongoing condition. Six to eight weeks may be typical, four if you're lucky, unless you're already a patient of a doctor who has publicized their availability. One may be a patient of, say, a willing surgeon but encounter resistance if the large health system's specialty clinic that the doctor is associated with doesn't consider you a patient of the clinic also.

Another potential delay relates to the drugs prescribed. Under Colorado's law, businesses and individuals may opt out in various ways. Individuals can morally and ethically object. Pharmacies may decline to stock the required substances. For certain formulations, a process known as compounding may be required; few pharmacies are "compounding pharmacies." A hidden snafu might also be a pharmacy's wholesale distributor that supplies a given retail location—if the distributor doesn't carry the drugs, the pharmacy cannot obtain them.

So the essential problem is that people mistakenly believe that MAID is casually available and accessible, anytime, anywhere. People wait too long to decide to seek MAID and risk failing to obtain it. In the case I was privy to, a 90-year-old dying person and their proxy had to endure, while seriously failing, multiple round trips across a large metropolitan area to meet with the doctors, apply, qualify, and obtain the prescriptions. They very nearly didn't make it—they very nearly landed in Failed dying.

Lastly, a medically-aided death is, in fact, a medical treatment requiring the full range of advocacy skills by proxies and family members: forecasting, knowledge, and supervision with as much diligence as for any other medical treatment.

Medical Professionals' Challenges in Providing Aided Dying

The other misapprehension that civilians are under is what it takes for medical professionals to engage in MAID. Engagement may be split into two aspects: administrative and technical.

Administratively, most doctors work with or for health systems, facilities, or large group practices which may, at the corporate level, decline to participate. Populations in rural areas served by a single system that opts out will need to go elsewhere to find willing doctors. For systems opting in, policies and procedures must be developed to govern how the system will manage, coordinate, and deliver aided dying. Since MAID is a profound paradigm shift, the people comprising the system may go through individual and collective soul-searching before opting in or out and before designing their policies and procedures. If you or your loved one are among the first applicants, expect to encounter confusion and uncertainty.

Doctors are not trained to purposely end life. This is apparent especially in the United States where, unlike British Columbia, Canada, euthanasia by injection is illegal; dying people must independently ingest the lethal agents (currently the only delivery method is oral; I am interested in but do not expect to see an intravenous method introduced in the United States). The laws do not require that physicians undergo any particular training. So doctors are on their own to assess each patient and, in consultation with colleagues and pharmacists as they see fit, to devise a reliable lethal "cocktail" on a case-by-case basis.

In the gentlest cases, death will be very quick—five to 15 minutes. Or, death could take five to 15 hours or even some days. We don't hear about longer deaths during legislative or election campaigns.

In the case I was privy to, the dying person's death took 11 hours. It was completely peaceful for the dying person but nerve-wracking for the attending adult child proxy. The hospice that they enrolled in was slow to assist and of limited help. Essentially, the two-person family was on its own.

Apparently, there's much for doctors to consider. Patients with many comorbidities may have an easier time dying than patients who are dying from one severe condition but whose bodies are otherwise strong. As a layperson, I'd express this by saying that a complete medical history needs to be known and understood at a deep level to maximize the chance for quick dying. There is no one-size-fits-all lethal agent.

For all these reasons, accessing aided dying is tough, most especially in the first year after each law takes effect. Perhaps surprisingly, these troubles persist even in jurisdictions like Oregon, now in its 21st year offering aided dying. Compared to another paradigm shift, it's ridiculously hard. In states where cannabis is now legal, adult residents can walk into any retail vendor and upon showing ID, immediately buy cannabis in many forms, walk out and drive home with their purchase. It is actually harder to find and obtain aided-dying services today than it was buying illegal cannabis from the 1970s to the 2010s. It seems to me that on a social scale both of these reforms represent deep change, are equally complex, and are managed very differently.

Lastly, my own reflection as one who worked to pass a law where I live and who has subsequently, if only tangentially, helped a dying person use it: dying and death is profound for all involved, a lesson that death literacy abundantly teaches. Dying in peace requires that we become hands-on involved. To do well, we must approach dying matters with humility and compassion as well as resolve.

— —

For people whose condition or timing make them ineligible for aided dying, Voluntarily Stopping Eating and Drinking (VSED) may be a viable pathway. Consult these books to learn more:
- *The Best Way to Say Goodbye*, Stanley Terman, MD, 2007, Life Transitions Publications
- *Choosing To Die*, Phyllis Shacter, 2017, PhyllisShacter.com

For people interested in personally directing their dying independent of the medico-legal system and societal norms, read the classic *Final Exit* by Derek Humphry.

Study Up, Make Some Sense:
Select Resources

Books Short List
- *My Mother, Your Mother: Embracing "Slow Medicine": The Compassionate Approach to Caring for your Aging Love Ones*, Dennis McCullough, MD, 2009, Harper.
- *Notes from the Waiting Room: Managing a Loved One's End-of-Life Hospitalization*, Bart Windrum, 2008, AxiomAction.
- *The Empowered Patient© Hospital Guide for Patients and Families* (free downloadable workbook), Julia Hallisy and Helen Haskell, 2008, EmpoweredPatientCoalition.org/patient-education.
- *The Art of Dying Well: A Practical Guide to a Good End of Life*, Katy Butler, scheduled for publication in 2019, Scribner.
- *The Five Invitations: Discovering What Death Can Teach Us About Living Fully*, Frank Ostaseski, 2017, Flatiron Books.

In the past, of the 100-plus books that I've read regarding end-of-life and medical matters, I've distilled my recommendations to three. They guide us and our surrogate advocates respectively from birds-eye level, mid-level, and ground-level. They are, in order: *My Mother, Your Mother*; *Notes from the Waiting Room*; and *The Empowered Patient© Hospital Guide for Patients and*

Families (a free download). *My Mother, Your Mother* describes the stages of decline and how to recognize them. *Notes from the Waiting Room* discusses unexamined aspects of engagement with medicine during hospitalizations. *The Empowered Patient Hospital Guide* is a tool for recording a loved one's hospital stay. Combined, these books stand as a go-to kit for understanding the phases of decline, orienting to and managing hospitalizations, and staying up-to-the-moment when hospitalized via a personally-kept chart (medical record).

I'm going out on a limb and adding a fourth book prior to its publication. It's due in 2019 and promises to address a wide range of practical matters pertaining to humane, well-supported late-stage lives and deaths. Katy Butler's first book, *Knocking on Heaven's Door: The Path to a Better Way of Death*, a memoir-reportage, established her as an end-of-life authority. Her forthcoming book, *The Art of Dying Well*, "covers navigating the medical territory from vigorous old age to death… boots-on-the-ground guidance, an emphasis on solutions and realistic medical decision-making… ways to give all the transitions of aging and loss their dignity… including the sacred, equally accessible to the religious, atheists, and free-range spiritualists."

Lastly, a new include to my expanded short list, from Buddhist teacher Frank Ostaseski, *The Five Invitations*. Although my work focuses on practical impediments to dying in peace, there's great value in upping our spiritual game. Buddhism offers a lot. I am not a participant; I've never been inclined toward rigorous practice but have long appreciated the few aspects of Buddhism that I'm aware of, especially clarity regarding the human condition. I summarize the value in one word: equanimity. Developing equanimity is the key, if not crucial, aspect for successful medical advocacy both for ourselves and as proxies for our loved ones. Equanimity can be cultivated. And we should all be busy tilling that soil; we'll need the shoots that sprout up for traction throughout our dying territory.

Online Shortlist: Facebook Groups

<u>Slow Medicine Facebook Group</u>   Katy Butler founded and curates the membership-only Slow Medicine with the help of member-administrators. Quite popular at over 4,000 members, the group manages to percolate as a daily resource of details, insights, and guidance. In addition to civilians, members include nurses, doctors, administrators, educators, and policy wonks deeply experienced across medical specialties. Katy's compassionate guiding hand serves as a model for participants' open engagement, making this internet forum a safe space. Inquisitiveness reigns freely; there seems to be no end of questions posed in the communal search to understand the forces shaping medical, late-life, and end-of-life experiences.

<u>To Die in Peace: Overcoming Obstacles Facebook Group</u>   I founded and curate this 700+ member group. It's relatively quiet, yet members report that they find value in what I, and occasionally others, post.

<u>Other Facebook Groups</u>   Creating peaceful conditions from, say, age 60 on up, especially regarding health, medical, and quality-of-life matters, is a varied pursuit spanning many aspects. Facebook seems to be, for better or worse, the platform where people congregate to share experiences and knowledge. Rather than list multiple groups here, I encourage you to search for key words and sample groups that turn up. In general, I prefer groups whose curation includes vetted membership over those groups that throw membership open to any and all comers.

Pricing Resource

ClearHealthCosts.com For U.S. residents: did you know that you can, and should, shop prices when contemplating undergoing medical tests and procedures? Clear Health Costs is Jeanne Pinder's project to obtain and publish comparative cash, government, and crowdsourced costs. Even if your area is not yet listed, perusing costs for included areas will be informative.

Appendix D
Matrix Visual History

For those interested in peeking behind the scenes: Windrum's Matrix of Dying Terms' initial development occurred over a three-month period. I worked in a spreadsheet because its cells offered a ready-made table. This is the spreadsheet file as I last left it in 2013:

		Windrum Early Twenty-first Century Western Dying Matrix			
	Living		**Dying**		**Vegetative**
		Onset	Progressed	Endstage	
Natural					
Self-directed	Suicide	Released	Dignified	Failed	
Medical		Early	Disguised	Endstate*	
Machine		Delayed	Indeterminate	Redundant	Vegetative
Matrix assumes no Death With Dignity statute				**includes palliative sedation*	
		Direct	Delayed	Denied	
			Disguised	De facto	
				Redundant	
Color Key	Legal or ethical	Illegal or unethical	by prevailing law/ethics		
Terms	Onset	(early) engaged, diseased, before disease limits ability			
	Progressed	(middle) passive, preliminary dying, disease progress may necessitate fami			
	Endstage	(late) incapacitated, end-stage dying			
	Self-directed	self-controlled under adverse condition; self-administered or family/friend			
	Machine	life support technology			

This was the early, ugly, and confusing graphic depiction of Windrum's Matrix:

Living		**Dying**			**Living Death**
		Onset	Progressed	Endstage	
	Control				
Accidental	World				
Suicidal	Self-Directed	Released	Dignified	Failed	
	Medical	Early	Midstream	Endstate	
	Machine	Delayed	Indeterminate	Redundant	Vegetative

This was the first formalized Matrix, circa 2013:

Non-terminal dying and Never* dying	Control	Dying		
		Onset	Progressed	Endstage
Accidental	World	Insleep		
SlowMotion	Medical	Early	Midstream	Endstate
Vegetative	Machine	Delayed	Indeterminate	Redundant
Suicidal	Personal	Released	Dignified	Failed

This was the first publicly shared Matrix, with 16 landings (on illuminated screens these green colors appear bright, even fluorescent):

Control	Abrupt Dying	Dying of natural disease			Never-ending Dying
		Onset	Progressed	Endstage	
World	Accidental	Insleep			
Medical	Erroneous	Early	Midstream	Endstate	SlowMo
Machine		Delayed	Indeterminate	Redundant	Vegetative
Personal	Suicidal	Released	Dignified	Failed	
Shared		Intentional	Palliative (comfort) and Hospice		

And, once again, the final Matrix of Dying Terms:

Windrum's Matrix of Dying Terms ™

Control	Abrupt Dying	Medically managed Dying			Never-ending Dying
		Onset	Progressed	Endstage	
World	Sudden	Insleep			SlowMotion
Medical	Erroneous	Early	Midstream	Endstate	
Machine	Emergency Room	Delayed	Suspended	Repetitive	Vegetative
Personal	Suicidal	Released	Postponed	Failed	
Shared		Collaborative			

LEGAL and/or ACCEPTED   ILLEGAL and/or UNACCEPTED   BOTH and/or AMBIGUOUS

The emblem for To Die in Peace: Overcoming Obstacles presents seven overlapping circles representing the interrelated obstacles to peaceful dying for which the program offers solutions. Transparency results in myriad color combinations, reflecting the complexity arising when we encounter obstacles to peaceful dying and the potential for balance when we succeed in living our end days peacefully:

Appendix E

The Quickie Button

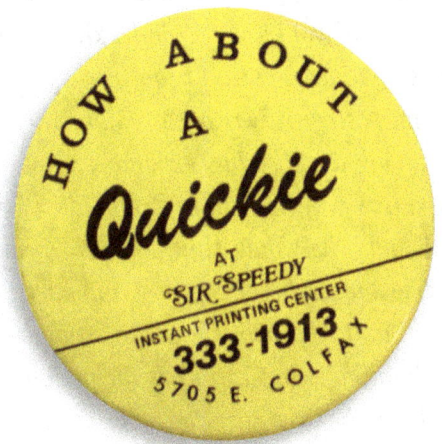

The Quickie button is real. Given the times we live in at this writing, I invite viewers to appreciate the Quickie button in the context of the 1970s and the playful spirit in which it was tendered to customers by the 50-something, mainstream parents of a hippie son (whose hippie attributes they disapproved). For me, the 2¼" button remains a precious and delightful connection to the years I worked alongside Mort and Ruth and to my memories of them as they successfully endeavored to realize the classic American Dream.

I have repurposed the Quickie button. I described how and why as I closed my 2013 TEDxFoCo talk, To Die in Peace: New Terms of Engagement:

One day, Dad walked in with a box of yellow buttons. He put that box on the edge of the counter. Whenever a customer would walk in the door—man, woman, or beast—he'd grab a button, he'd go out to greet them, and he'd pop 'em the question. That question was out of bounds, but Mom let him get away with it, I looked on with astonishment—and sometimes jealousy—and the customers had a good time.

You probably get the idea that I ask a lot of questions.... Among them is 'what would the folks think of what I do and what I say since they died?' I think Mom would say 'I don't know about that Rap...'. I think Dad would say 'I had no idea I bequeathed you that button. And I understand its repurposing. It was out of bounds when I asked it but over the years our dying territory has expanded so much that now this question, asked in a new way, is right in the middle of the ball field.'

I think if Dad could, he would shuffle on out here with his walker and that grin, and he'd reach into his pocket and back 38 years and he'd hold out the button, and he'd pop you the question: 'Would you like a Quickie?' It's shorthand for what I think is the profound question of our age: Is protracted dying the necessary cost of extended living?

Who owns your dying? Who controls? What is required of you, and of me, to die in peace? I think the obstacles, the impediments, are so many, so huge, so rapid, and so weighty in their result as to require from all of us acts of citizenship.

So I say 'Study Up, make some sense of 21st century impediments. Time to grow up before we grow old.'

Want to die at peace? Got to die in peace. Reiner Maria Rilke, the 20th century poet, said it beautifully and succinctly in his masterwork, *The Sonnets to Orpheus: Be Ahead of All Parting*. Be ahead of all parting. Yes, it's a challenge, but guess what? You're young—or young at heart; we've got the time and we can do it.

It's up to each of us, and all of us, to change this paradigm.

Appendix F

Coming In and Speaking Out

I am available for keynote and plenary speeches on the material covered in *The Promised Landing*. I include a shortened guided group recitation covering several dying territory landings so that your audience may experience the alchemy that occurs when cognition transmutes to feeling through the unusual power of group recitation. I'm always on the lookout for a reason to perform the Never Say Die Rap, so its inclusion is possible, if not likely. And given the opportunity, I love to block additional time to conduct a workshop at events where I speak.

Our Dying Territory workshops cover everything in chapters 1–9, including the full group recitation. Allow three hours, or two hours for a shortened version.

To Die in Peace: Overcoming Obstacles is an eight-hour workshop. The first several hours, of an afternoon or evening, are devoted to Our Dying Territory and the full experience of Windrum's Matrix of Dying Terms. Subsequent hours delve into the other six obstacles and what we can do to mitigate or overcome them.

Bart Windrum
AxiomAction.com
Bart@AxiomAction.com

Acknowledgments

Jennifer Ballentine Deep thanks to Jennifer, president of the end-of-life consultancy The Iris Project and, as of September 2017, Executive Director of the California State University San Marcos Institute of Palliative Care. Jennifer was the person I turned to upon receiving the unbidden "zillion words for snow" message, and she suggested early on, over lunch in Denver's Highlands neighborhood, that I include a landing for dying within the purview of hospice services. Jennifer and I had unexpectedly reconnected in the end-of-life space approximately 20 years after our last prior contact; I had supplied graphic design services to her and husband's book composition business. Thank you Jennifer for your consistent encouragement of the Matrix and for championing my end-of-life work over the years.

Dave deBronkart Internationally recognized as a patient-rights evangelist, Dave deBronkart ("ePatient Dave") gave me an incomparable gift early after I'd developed the Matrix. With curiosity, allegiance to data integrity, and marketing smarts, Dave took the early, clumsily-designed Matrix home with him from where we met at Regina Holliday's first Partnership With Patients conference, studied it with scant description from me (at his own request!), and through email engaged in a spirited discussion of what he thought it was and how I might improve it. Dave's insights helped me refine the Matrix layout—a huge contribution as the early layout was a mess. Dave also clued me that null values are meaningful, occupying space of equal importance with other values. And he suggested branding the work as "Windrum's Matrix." For all this, my ongoing gratitude, Dave.

Kim Mooney This book would likely not exist were it not for Kim, a veteran of the Boulder, Colorado end-of-life scene who now runs Practically Dying, an education and advance planning consultancy. Kim's everywhere like the ether, and I don't recall when or how we met. Periodically we'd lunch, and I'd share my evolving work with her. After what must have been a decade she took a more active interest in what I was doing. When I later asked what changed, she replied that I wasn't nearly as angry about it all as I had been for many years. In late 2014 Kim suggested that we conduct a focus group session on my lexicon. With her extensive contacts plus mine we convened a group of medical professionals and highly informed lay people from Boulder's civilian end-of-life reform community. The session occurred in March 2015. It was there and then that the significance of Windrum's Matrix began to evidence itself. For actively welcoming me as an end-of-life peer, my appreciation, Kim.

Terry Kori Terry, a lifelong friend with unique perception, once set me on a bit of a cat and mouse search for meaning hidden in plain sight within a business-builder reality show series. The lesson had to do with the losses inherent in turning away expert assistance when fortunate enough to have it at hand and, therefore, the value to be gained by seeking assistance. That message took root and over some years it led to the aforementioned focus group. The openness required to attract that then led, over more years, to a behavioral leap: my development and inclusion of the guided group recitation during presentations of Our Dying Territory / Windrum's Matrix of Dying Terms. Conducting the recitation is a stretch for me, and I perceive its value as profound for those studying this material. For helping me help others to use all our perceptive abilities to better become death literate, enormous thanks, Terry.

Katy Butler   Katy, author of *Knocking on Heaven's Door: The Path to a Better Way of Death*, coined the term "misadventure" to create an umbrella under which to distinguish dangerous medical snafus from erroneous ones. She also suggested the addition of an emergency room landing to account for abrupt deaths within that unique milieu. Thank you Katy for cross-pollinating as we each develop and refine our respective end-of-life lexicons. Compadre, indeed.

James Leonard Park   James, an existential philosopher and curator of several Facebook groups devoted to right-to-die matters, has written extensively on medical ethics, death, and dying including an especially deep look at what I call self-directed dying. Thanks, James, for suggesting that I replace "indeterminate" with "suspended," a term more easily understandable by people who don't spend as much time musing about these matters as we do.

Nick Armstrong   Nick, former curator of TEDx events in Fort Collins, Colorado, took a chance when accepting my proposal to present at TEDxFoCo 2013; when he asked if I was serious with my end-of-life talk proposal, I waxed so strongly that he figured I was. The Matrix wound up occupying one-third of the talk. Developing and delivering a TED-style talk upped my game and began an ongoing process of refining how I introduce Windrum's Matrix to the world. Having the talk filmed and posted online magnifies my reach. And, as serendipity would have it, the Never Say Die Rap likely would not otherwise exist; it arose as an outlet for the frustration inherent in end-of-life reform coupled with the intense focus required of TEDx talk preparation. Nick, I continue to appreciate the opportunity you provided.

Deborah Fink Windrum Deborah, my wife of thirty years, served as this book's early and final editor. Her sharp observations and rejection, through overexposure, of my writing idiosyncrasies helped me to finally make sense. Although she wasn't "on the ground" with my sister Judy and I during our parents' demises, she's had a ringside seat throughout the emergence of my end-of-life lexicon. In particular, her periodic befuddlement over the Matrix has been useful—if I couldn't explain it in a way to make this smart lady understand, I knew I needed to keep refining my presentation. Deborah, thank you for putting up with endless morbid conversation, both upbeat and down.

Ruth Hanna Logue Greenberg and Morton Greenberg
These good-hearted people raised me with minimal judgment, providing maximum latitude and crucial assists at key times throughout our lives. Their end-of-life landings, about which I have been unendingly regretful, have inadvertently given birth to this body of work, my end-of-life lexicon. I have envisioned the state of being necessary to bring this lexicon forth as standing on a cold dock in thick fog holding the rusted chain of a hulking ship floating on deep waters in a narrow location. The ship represented my parents and my memory of them; the chain, the connection I had to maintain in order to develop my thoughts; the fog, the emotional aspect such persistent connection precipitated; and the constricted environs the solitary construct in which my agitation and restlessness produced this work. Perhaps, with the completion of this book, I will lay down the rusted chain; I'm unsure that I have any new insights to add. If so, then I must turn away and bid my parents a second goodbye, most consciously and bittersweet. I have held the chain willfully—and willingly—for fourteen years and might feel adrift without its weight. We cannot see through the fog at life's edge and may only hope that our loved ones' souls are at peace no matter where and how they landed. May my parents' memory

live further on should this end-of-life lexicon prove useful beyond satisfying my own queries.

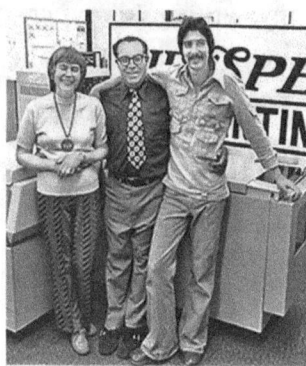 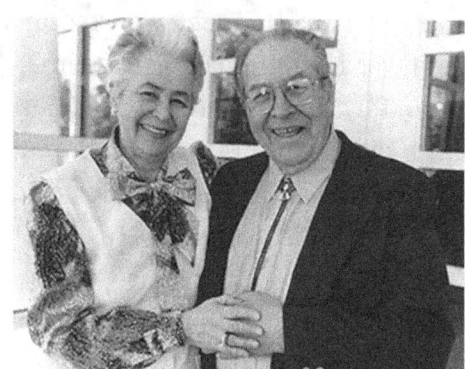

— —

Thanks to front section and rear section reader Jennifer Ballentine who encouraged me not to over-refine over my voice in the former and fact-checked details in the latter.

Vignette reader and 2015 focus group participant Claire Riley RN stimulated a deepened query into the intersection of fatal nosocomial MRSA infection and medical error (which nonetheless didn't change my, and many others', assessment that they are one and the same).

Early manuscript readers had the rough task of reading a rough manuscript. What evidence I had from the feedback I received indicated that they didn't make it all the way, a circumstance I decided to own. Each reported aspects of the writing (er, thinking!) that stymied their ability to connect. Thanks to Carla Berg, Lee Tilson, and Ptarmigan Emory for providing spot-on insights that resulted in crucial refinement of the front sections over months of subsequent, challenging rewrites, ultimately leading to a "zero mouse buttons" organizational solution.

Second-round manuscript readers had it better with a fairly refined manuscript to read. Lisa Ahbel, Jim Bates, and Bob Kenny offered good, great, and greater input that stimulated me to significantly improve this book.

In all cases, I took seriously every critique, especially sticking points, and have done my best to address them in what I hope has been a successful attempt to welcome the widest variety of readers given the demanding nature of this topic and the bar I have set.

For the first time I publicly exposed my graphic design process, via my personal Facebook page, inviting comments and informal voting for several cover designs and their refinement. Thanks to those who commented, for adding some experiential texture to the persnickety and always gratifying-in-the-end graphic design process.

Bette Frick's copyediting helped polish this book's core pages; any remaining deviations from publishing norms are mine.

A shout-out goes to Reina Callier, Ph.D at the University of Colorado at Boulder Classics department for graciously refining my attempt at a Latin translation for the Opaque Dying Marketplace: *Opacum Emporium Mortis*. The example for Latinizing phrases that medicine overlooks was set by patient-advocate Joel Selmeier, who devised a Latin term for medical error: *Nequamitis*. I agree with Joel that using Latin, the language of medicine, helps underscore the seriousness of medical shortcomings that induce deleterious effects on individuals, families, and society.

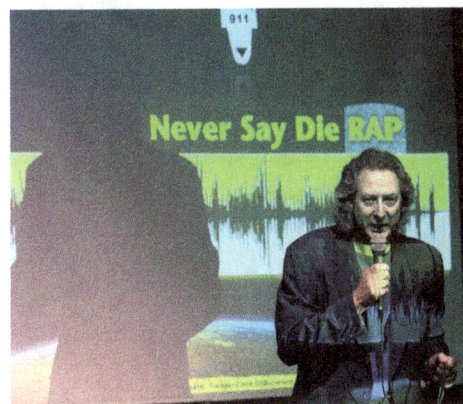
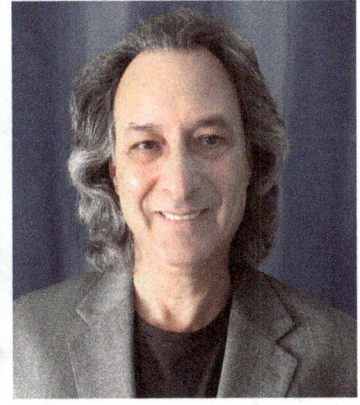

Bart Windrum

Index

A
Advocating medically 178
    advance directives, list 180–185
    calling 911 185
    medical aid in dying 192
    medical approaches 187
    select resources 198
    taproot 178

C
Cardinal Aspects 44
    Control 46
    Time 45
Care (+ various suffixes) 14, 16, 26–27, 31, 138, 162, 178–180

D
Demises as destinations 11
    way stations 6, 24, 30, 52–53, 58, 77, 83, 102, 138

G
Gateway 3, 5–8, 29, 102
Glossary of terms 29

H
Heroics 131

L
Landings 56
    Collaborative 76
    Delayed 69
    Early 65
    Emergency Room 63
    Endstate 67
    Erroneous 61
    Failed 75
    Insleep 59
    Midstream 66
    Postponed 74
    Released 73
    Repetitive 71
    SlowMotion 68
    Sudden 60
    Suicidal 64
    Suspended 70
    Vegetative 72

M
Matrix. *See* **Windrum's Matrix**
    definitions 29
Medical Approaches 187
    Choosing Wisely 190
    geriatric medicine 187
    hospice 188
    palliative care 188
    Right Care 190
    Slow Medicine 189
Medical error 139

N
Never Say Die Rap 176
    lyrics applied
        call 911 when it's
            time to pass 185
        can't touch the sky 180
        chart your glide path 4
        don't mean to be mean 151
        if you don't talk
            you don't get no say 187
        independent thinker,
            no one's rube 178
        no bro ma'am you
            ain't goin' nowhere 192
        study up, make some sense 198
        want to die at peace,
            got to die in peace 36

O

Obstacles 125
  all obstacles, list 128
  difficulty distinguishing
    among dying situations 130
  exposure to medical snafus 139
  ignorance regarding
    life-support matters 141
  inability to advocate medically 145
  obstacles 1-3 reflection 137
  obstacles 4-6 reflection 147
  Opaque Dying Marketplace 149
  Our Rights of Passage 126
  over-reliance on
    advance directives 134
  recap of obstacles 167
  trouble determining
    when enough is enough 131
Opaque Dying Marketplace 149
Our dying territory (key thoughts)
  3, 6–7, 10, 21, 25, 27, 29, 38, 44,
  49, 51, 58, 77, 83, 102, 126, 130,
  138, 160, 171, 199

P

Pain 23
  extrinsic, intrinsic, promise 23–24
Peace, getting to 7
Poems 174
  Never Say Die Rap 176
  Sweating Oil 175
Practicalities 34
  advance directives, surrogates 34
  die in peace, die at peace 36
  spiritual engagement 36
  end-of-life management
    tripod 35, 128
Promises
  consideration 9, 23–27, 34, 37–38

Q

Quickie button 205

R

Recitation 102
  audio file 103
  rationale 6, 22, 55, 102
  Collaborative 121
  Delayed 114
  Early 110
  Emergency Room 108
  Endstate 112
  Erroneous 107
  Failed 120
  Insleep 105
  Midstream 111
  Peaceful 123
  Peace-less 122
  Postponed 119
  Released 118
  Repetitive 116
  SlowMotion 113
  Sudden 106
  Suicidal 109
  Suspended 115
  Vegetative 117
Rusted Gate 174
  poem 175
  reference 8

S

Situations (consideration) 3, 5,
  10, 14, 20–22, 24, 25, 26, 29, 30,
  31, 32, 36–37, 40–41, 44, 48–49,
  50–51, 54, 56–58, 77, 124, 167
Speaking, by author 207

T
To Die in Peace:
  Our Rights of Passage 125
Tripod, end-of-life 35, 128, 172
21st century end-of-life milieu 172

V
Vignettes 83
  Collaborative 101
  Delayed 94
  Early 90
  Emergency Room 88
  Endstate 92
  Erroneous 87
  Failed 100
  Insleep 85
  Midstream 91
  Postponed 99
  Released 98
  Repetitive 96
  SlowMotion 93
  Sudden 86
  Suicidal 89
  Suspended 95
  Vegetative 97

W
Why 1
  death literacy 8
  dying situations 41
  equanimity and resolve 37
  foresee and consider 20
  likelihoods 9
  map our dying territory 25
  much smarter 26–27
  promise pain 24
  unambiguous assessment 38
  working voyage 10
Windrum's Matrix of Dying Terms 33
  aspects 52
  cardinal aspects 44
  dying territory 50
  ethics and legalities 78
  genesis 39
  landings 56
  neutrality 54
  vignettes 83

www.ingramcontent.com/pod-product-compliance
Lightning Source LLC
Chambersburg PA
CBHW052019290426
44112CB00014B/2302